THE BODY SCULPTING BIBLE FOR

CHEST & ARMS

THE BODY SCULPTING BIBLE FOR

CHEST & ARMS

James Villepigue

Hugo Rivera

Photography by
Peter Field Peck

healthyliving**books**

New York • London

www.bodysculptingbible.com

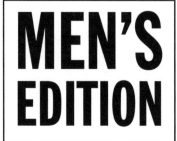

MEN'S EDITION

A Healthy Living Book
Published by Hatherleigh Press
5–22 46th Avenue, Suite 200
Long Island City, NY 11101
www.hatherleighpress.com

Villepigue, James C.
The body sculpting bible for chest & arms : men's edition / by James Villepigue.
p. cm.
ISBN 1–57826–212–7
1. Bodybuilding. 2. Exercise for men. I. Title.
 GV546.5.V534 2004
 613.7'1885—dc22
2005021994

Seek the advice of your physician before starting any physical fitness program.

Healthy Living Books are available for bulk purchase, special promotions, and premiums. For information on reselling and special purchase opportunities, please call us at 1–800–528–2550 and ask for the Special Sales Manager.

Special thanks to RoseMarie Alfieri.

Cover Designed by Deborah Miller
Interior design by Deborah Miller and Michael Wood

10 9 8 7 6 5 4 3 2 1
Printed in Canada

Dedication

I would like to dedicate this exciting project to the most important people in my life. To my mom, Nancy, a genuine angel on Earth: I am truly blessed by God to be your son and I simply adore you. To my beautiful and talented sister, Debbie, aka Deborah: My love for you could never cease and I am, as I have always said, "So very proud of you!" To my awesome Dad, Jim: I love you more than you could ever know. I miss you so much pal. Thank you for helping me to become the man I am...Warrior Overwhelmed...I love you, I adore you, and I honor you every moment of my life. God bless you, pal! To God, thank you, thank you, thank you! To my Fiancée Heather: Thank you again for all of your incredible and much needed support. I love you and look forward to our wonderful life together. To all of my beautiful family, loved ones, and friends: You all know who you are and I love you all very much!

Finally, to all of you reading, I owe a great debt of gratitude to you all. Thank you so very much for your interest in our work. We truly hope you enjoy. Believe and achieve. God bless!

James

Dedication

First of all, I would like to thank God for giving me the talent and the ability to not only be a writer, but also for allowing me to make a living doing what I love.

Having said that, I would like to dedicate this book to my number one fans and biggest supporters in the world, my lovely wife Lina and my son Chad. I could not be anywhere near where I am today if it would not be for your love and support Lina. From the bottom of my heart, thank you so much for everything you have ever done for me. Chad, by seeing how hard you work in school and how industrious you are, you inspire me to be even better every day; thanks so much pal.

I also want to dedicate this book to my parents Haydeé and Arturo, my grandparents Nydia and Dr. Raul Rivera, and my great grandmother María Mercedes in Puerto Rico, who have always supported me from the day I was born and who ensured that I always had what I needed in order to be successful. Also, for instilling in me the belief that if you put your mind to it you can accomplish anything. Also, to my brothers Raul and Javier Rivera for their support and encouragement. In addition, I want to dedicate this book to my in-laws Edith and Alvaro, who have always treated me as their own son and who have supported my endeavors in every way, shape or form possible.

I want to also give thanks to my co-author and great friend James Villepigue, for without his help, I could not be where I am today either. Jimmy, you are a great human being and an awesome friend. To my good friend William Kemp for all of his faith in me and superb advice. Bill, it is a true honor to know you and I thank you for all you have ever done for me. Always thanks to Dave and Laree Draper, for their help in introducing me to this great industry. To Stella Juarez, author of Stella's Kitchen, for her support, friendship, and for motivating me to apply to become the new www.bodybuilding.about.com guide. To Brian Ward who is one of the best friends anyone can have. Brian, I cannot thank you enough for all the support you have given me in these past few years. You're the man. To Peter Peck, who is the most talented and passionate photographer I have ever known. Without you, Peter, the books would only be half complete. To everyone at Hatherleigh, Andrew, Kevin, Andrea, Alyssa, Deborah, Erin, RoseMarie and everyone else that helps make these publications possible, a big thank you! And last but certainly not least, to my fans and avid readers who at the end of the day are the only reason that I exist. Thank you so much for all your support and please know that I am here to help you achieve all your fitness goals.

All the best!
Hugo

Table of Contents

INTRODUCTION

Build a Chiseled Chest and Awesome Arms 1

PART I: GO FOR IT

CHAPTER 1: Your Upper Body Muscles 7

CHAPTER 2: Fitness Fuel 21

PART II: THE EXERCISES

CHAPTER 3: Ultimate Stretching 33

CHAPTER 4: Chest 45

CHAPTER 5: Back and Shoulders 61

CHAPTER 6: Biceps and Triceps 93

CHAPTER 7: The Core 125

PART III: THE WORKOUTS

CHAPTER 8: Beginner Workout 145

CHAPTER 9: Intermediate Workout 155

CHAPTER 10: Advanced Workout 163

APPENDIX A: TRAINING JOURNAL .170

APPENDIX B: FOOD CHARTS AND NUTRITION 172

Precautions

You should always consult a physician before starting any weight gain or fat reduction training/nutrition program.

A basic metabolic test, thyroid, lipid and testosterone panel is recommended prior to starting this program in order to detect anything that can prevent you from making the most out of your efforts.

Consult your doctor regarding these tests.

If you are unfamiliar with any of the exercises, consult an experienced trainer to instruct you on the proper form and execution of the unfamiliar exercise. Improper form can lead to injury.

The instructions and advice presented herein are not intended as a substitute for medical or other personal professional counseling.

HR Fitness Inc., From Fat to Phat Publishing, Inc., and the editors and authors disclaim any liability or loss in connection with the use of this system, its programs, and advice herein.

Introduction
Build a Chiseled Chest and Awesome Arms

When we wrote the original *Body Sculpting Bible for Men* books, our goal was to provide guys with a comprehensive whole–body workout program based on proven methods of training that we've used with our clients with great success. The response to the book has been fabulous and we are grateful to all who have found the book helpful in their quest for a healthy, fit, sculpted body.

Readers also have shared their opinions about the book and offered suggestions for the future. This book is a result of your suggestions; namely that you are particularly concerned about sculpting and building your chest and arms. This is not surprising to us: our male clients often want to increase their chest and biceps muscles and, once again, we are ready to deliver the

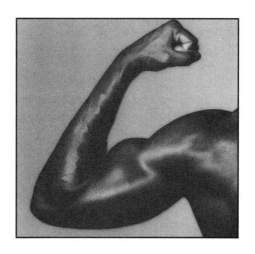

THE **BODY SCULPTING BIBLE** FOR
CHEST & ARMS

goods. Let's think about why so many men are concerned with developing these two body parts. The salient reason, of course, is that your chest and arms are two very exposed, visible parts of your body. You've probably noticed a fit–looking guy wearing a tank top, or cut–off shirt, with noticeably muscular and well–defined arms and a massive chest and said to yourself, "Wow, that dude is in good shape."

The truth is that you really can't determine whether he's truly in good shape or if it's just his arms and chest that are well built and defined. True, those two body parts may look great, but what about the rest of his body? Is his back strong? Are his abdominals trained? For this reason training your whole body is important, and the Chest & Arms Workout is just one component of a full fitness regimen.

That said, while on your journey toward achieving your fitness goals, there's nothing wrong with letting everyone think that you already are in great shape. Science tells us our sub–conscious mind cannot differentiate between fact and fiction. When you act as if you are already in great shape, you will work hard to make it become a reality.

Let's face it. There are no quick fixes to creating a naturally great–looking body. But, in a world obsessed with vanity, why shouldn't you send a message of confidence during your quest?

Consider this; you will reach your overall fitness goals soon enough, so by all means live as if your goals have already come true.

In the *Body Sculpting Bible Chest & Arms*, we present an upper body workout program that homes in on the muscles you most want to sculpt, and that stresses balance between opposing muscle groups. The three- to four–day–a–week workouts are designed to elicit a defined, strong upper body using the 14–day periodization training technique that we introduced in the original *Body Sculpting Bible*. These workouts can be done as stand–alone programs, or as adjuncts to the workouts in the *Body Sculpting Bible*.

This book begins with an overview of your upper body, including a description of the upper body anatomy and kinesiology (a study of body movements), so that you can understand how your upper body muscles were designed to function. We then go into the specifics of weight training and the Chest & Arms Workout, providing you with the information you'll need to engage in the workout program safely and effectively. In Chapter Two, we present a nutritional program that will maximize your body's muscle–building potential. As with the training program, we believe strongly in a balanced approach to nutrition— one that doesn't demonize any nutrient and which provides energy via consumption of nutrient–dense foods. In Chapter Three you'll find information on stretching, and a sample stretch program for all of the muscles covered in the Chest & Arms Workout.

Part II of the book presents detailed descriptions of each of the exercises, along with tips from us on how to modify the exercises for progression and safety. The workout programs—Beginner (8 weeks), Intermediate, and Advanced (6 weeks)—follow. All are designed to keep your body challenged throughout the given time period, based on your individual fitness level.

We hope you enjoy the workouts we created for your upper body. As you begin the program, bear in mind that while this workout focuses on your upper body for a period of time, it does not replace performing exercises for all of your body's muscles. It is important to train your entire body and to incorporate cardiovascular training a few times a week, either on your off days or after your sculpting workouts. In the next chapter we explain how you can incorporate this regimen into a whole–body training routine, so that you achieve your upper–body goals without sacrificing the rest of your fitness needs.

Having said that, let's get started!

Part I

Go For It

You want a chest that's chiseled, one that commands attention and admiration. You want arms that are awesome—strong, sculpted, serious arms. You want not only to look great, but to feel great, too. Go for it. Here in Part I we talk about what it takes to build your chest and arms. You'll learn about the muscles in your upper body—how they work and interact with each other. You'll also learn how to fuel your body with nutrient–dense foods in order to maximize both your health and your fitness gains.

THE BODY SCULPTING BIBLE FOR CHEST & ARMS

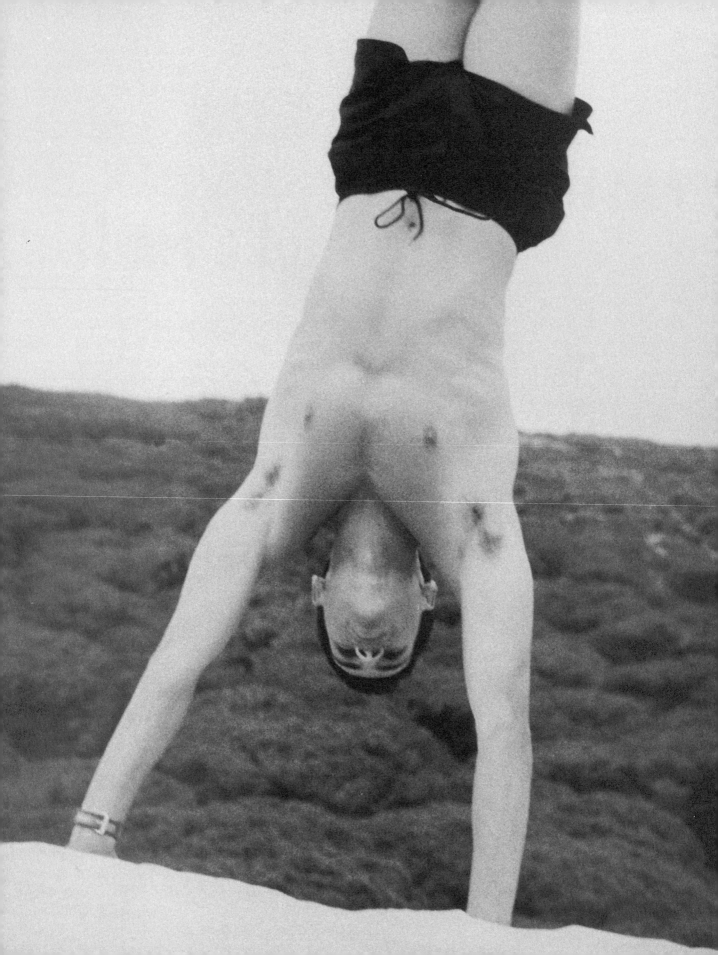

Chapter 1
Your Upper Body Muscles

To build an amazing upper body you need to have some understanding of the muscles in the chest, arms, and back, and how they function. This chapter goes into some basics of anatomy and kinesiology, before discussing the specifics of your Chest & Arms Workout protocol.

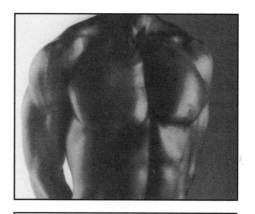

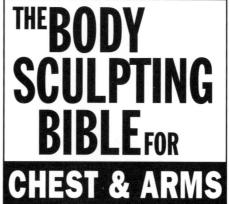

1

THE CHEST & ARMS

The Chest & Arms Workout homes in on the major muscles of your upper body to give you a strong, well–defined chest and ripped arms. In particular, it works the muscles of the chest: the pectoralis major and minor, and the two major muscle groups in the arms: the two–headed biceps and the three–headed triceps.

A LESSON ON ANATOMY AND KINESIOLOGY

The pectoral muscles help bring your arms together by flexing and rotating your shoulders in toward your body. The biceps, which consist of a long–head and short–head muscle, are located in the fronts of your arms between your shoulder and your inside elbow. The biceps flex your arms by bringing your wrist closer to your shoulder. They also turn or rotate the forearm, so that the palm of the hand faces up; this is called supination. The triceps, a three–headed muscle located at the back of the shoulder and running down the rear of the upper arm, extends your elbows. Because the biceps' primary function is arm flexion (bringing the forearms towards the shoulders) and the triceps' is arm extension (moving the forearm away from the shoulders), they are opposing muscle groups.

When you work the larger muscle groups of the upper body, you also work the smaller muscles. For example, when performing a push up, you are not only working your pectoralis muscles in the chest, but also training your triceps and shoulders, which act as sec-ondary helper or assisting muscles. Likewise, when you train the major muscles in your back, such as the lats, you also involve the shoulders and biceps (the muscles of the back and shoulder also are discussed below in the balance section).

For this reason, it is generally recommended to work the larger muscle groups first in a given workout session. Otherwise, you will tire the helper muscles out and they will not be able to work as effectively when you perform your lat pulldown or chest press.

EXERCISES TO CHISEL THE CHEST

There are a wide variety of exercises that target the pectoral major and minor muscles. For instance, you have incline, flat and decline bench presses that can be performed with dumbbells or barbells. You also have exercises like chest dips, push–ups, incline push–ups, dumbbell pullovers and incline, flat and decline flyes. To achieve a fully balanced and well defined chest, it is important to take advantage of the several exercises and angles available to you.

It's easy to get into an exercise rut. This can occur when you continue to do the same exercises, with no change in the exercise itself or the order in which you perform them. The problem with this approach is that you are always recruiting the same muscle fibers, in the same ways, resulting in limited gains of muscle, strength, and definition. In addition, once your nervous system gets used to an exercise and a specific repetition range, the next time the routine is repeated, your body will recruit even fewer muscle fibers. As you can see, this will lead to a pattern that yields zero results.

In a nutshell, it's all about challenging your body. To consistently see new and improved results, you must trick your nervous system and shock the muscles into growth. The next time you work out, perform your exercises by altering each of the angles at which you perform them. For example, instead of doing a standard preacher curl, where the angle of the upper arms is on a diagonal plane, turn the top of the preacher pad around, so that the angle of the upper arm will now be on a vertical plane (straight up and down).

This change in the angle will recruit different muscle fibers, thereby greatly increasing muscle stimulation and results! Another example is the fly, which involves bringing your arms together, toward the center of your chest (adducting your arms). You can perform the fly on a flat bench, a decline bench, or an incline bench to vary the area of emphasis. If you use an incline bench, the upper muscles will be accentuated whereas if you use a decline bench the emphasis will be greater in the lower chest. The push–up is yet another example. You can perform a push–up flat on the floor; with your arms on a bench (incline push–up) or fitness ball; or with your feet on a bench or ball and your arms on the floor (decline push–up).

Other ways to add variety with the same exercise is to alternate using machines and free weights and to add balance components (perform an exercise with a stability ball or balance board). In your Chest & Arms Workout you'll find that we use all of the variations described above. These variations, combined with the powerful 14–Day Periodization Principles, in which sets, repetitions, and rest in between sets are constantly changed, will provide a sure–fire way to get results fast!

EXERCISES TO BUILD THE ARMS

The biceps and triceps muscles, located in the front and back of your arms, are the major arm muscles we focus on in the Chest & Arms Workout. Since the biceps work to flex the arms, the exercises involve biceps curls at varying angles and positions—for example, Curl (Arms Turned Out). There is the preacher curl, which is a great isolation exercise since you use a special bench, or incline bench, to lean into the curl; and a dumbbell curl, which adds a balance challenge. The basic triceps exercises all involve extending the forearms while keeping the upper arms (from the shoulder to the elbows) stationary. You'll find a number of variations, including the kickback, pushdown, and triceps dips to ensure that you target all three heads of the triceps for maximum mass and definition.

ALL ABOUT BALANCE

While this book's purpose is to help you achieve a chiseled chest and awesome arms, one really important concept we want to stress is the importance of equally training opposing muscle groups. The back and chest are opposing muscle groups, as are the biceps and triceps. Training opposing muscles is vital in order to achieve balance and prevent injury that occurs when one muscle group is strong and the opposite is weak. In men, we often see this situation when it comes to the chest and back.

In general, men want a well–defined, muscular chest and large arms; consequently, this is where they focus their training, often neglecting to also train their back muscles. The result is an overly rounded front, and propensity for back pain and injury. And on a purely aesthetic basis, even though you cannot see your back with your shirt on, when you're out on the beach or going shirtless in the summer, your back is visible for all to see. Wouldn't you rather have a sculpted back that complements your defined chest, rather than one that looks like your chest's anemic brother?

Another frequent area of neglect is the shoulders. Despite the fact you train the fronts of the shoulders when you train your chest, it is of utmost importance to also target the shoulders' side and rear heads, not only to prevent strength imbalances that can lead to shoulder injury, but also to create a nice tri–dimensional look. A physique that exhibits a great chest and arms, but lacks shoulder and back development is imbalanced. Your goals in creating a great body should include building muscle symmetry (balance). This not only makes a body look great, but also helps to prevent muscle injuries.

Now that we've established the importance of not ignoring the back and shoulders, let's look at their anatomical function. The main back muscles are the latissimus dorsi, trapezius, rhomboids, and erector spinae. The latissimus dorsi (lats) muscles extend your arms, bring your shoulders together behind your body, and internally rotate your arms; the trapezius raises and moves your shoulders; the rhomboids elevate and rotate the scapula (the triangular bones at the backs of your shoulders); the erector spinae are the chief flexors of the vertebral column.

The shoulder is your body's most mobile joint and involves the action of several major muscles. While your back and chest muscles act on the shoulder, the deltoid muscles are located on the shoulder itself. They are triangular muscles and include three sections: the anterior deltoid (or front shoulder) muscles flex and rotate your arm. The mid-deltoid (or side shoulder) muscles abduct your arm; in other words, they move it away from your body. Finally, the posterior deltoid (or rear shoulder) muscles extend your arm and also rotate it externally.

The other group of shoulder muscles is the rotator cuff muscles, which work very much like a circus tent, to balance one another. The rotator cuff consists of four small muscles, stabilizers and movers that surround the scapula. These muscles, starting from the top one on the scapula and going clockwise, are called the supraspinatus, the infraspinatus, the teres minor and the subscapularis. Because of this, this group of muscles is often called the SITS muscle. These muscles attach to your upper arm (humerus) and externally and internally rotate and abduct (move away from the torso) the shoulder. They are often neglected in a training regimen. Over the long term, this causes a strength imbalance, because as the shoulder gets stronger, the rotator cuff muscles get weaker, if not trained. Ultimately, this can lead to rotator cuff injuries, a very common malady for people who bench press impressive amounts of weights, but neglect to train their rotators. You do not need to use heavy weight to train the rotator cuff muscles. In fact, if you use too heavy a weight, you risk injuring them. Training with the proper amount of weight is essential. Exercises for the back and shoulders, along with detailed descriptions, are found in Chapter Five.

ABDOMINAL AND CORE TRAINING

In addition to the upper extremity muscles, this book features a workout for the muscles of your abdominals, pelvis and lower back (your body's core).

There are four main muscle groups that make up the full abdominal wall.

- the rectus abdominis (composed of upper and lower abdominals)
- the oblique muscles
- the intercostal muscles
- the serratus anterior

RECTUS ABDOMINIS—THE PRIMARY ABDOMINAL MUSCLES

The muscle that extends from the top of the pelvis to the sternum is called the rectus abdominis. This is the primary abdominal muscle, which when properly developed (assuming that the person has low enough body fat levels) gives the illusion of a six–pack. Its function is to pull the upper torso towards the hips when the body is only slightly flexed at the waist. This is the reason why when performing a sit–up, any additional torso movement done past the initial 30 degrees from the floor will not stimulate the abs; instead the hips will complete the movement. Therefore partial sit–ups, performed with the torso moving up to 30 degrees, and crunches are great allies in the quest to achieve great abs.

However, if you really want to maximally stimulate the abdominals, prevent lower back problems and get the most "bang for your buck," you need to also consider that the anatomy of the rectus abdominis requires you to bend your torso backward by 15 to 20 degrees, in order to fully reach these muscles' greatest potential.

Consider this: training the abs on the floor will only provide a flat surface. This not only prevents your abs from receiving maximal stimulation, but it also does not allow you to properly engage, contract, and protect your lower back for times when your body is bent backward (as is often the case when advanced bodybuilders perform exercises like standing military presses).

The best solution is to purchase a fitness

ball (also called a Swiss ball). A fitness ball is a great investment (they only run about $15 to $45). It will allow you to get the necessary backward bend to maximally stimulate your abs.

Overall, crunches performed on a fitness ball are your best bet for a maximally developed midsection.

Since the rectus abdominis also have muscles located in the lower region, which help maintain proper postural alignment, it is recommended to include reverse crunches performed on the fitness ball (for proper balance and safety, please make sure that you hold onto a stationary, sturdy object when performing this movement) as this exercise will allow you to go below the neutral (flat) position.

Oblique Muscles Function and Exercises

The external obliques are the muscles at the sides of the waist. The external obliques are multifaceted, consisting of three layers of muscles: the internal obliques, the transverse obliques, and external obliques. Together, these muscles contract to tilt the torso, as well as twist it, from side to side. While you would not want to build massive obliques (this would take away from symmetry and give the illusion of a thick waist), these muscles do need to be trained in order to maintain ideal postural alignment.

A great exercise for the obliques is the Twist on the Ball, performed on a fitness ball. It exercises the muscles' rotating capabilities.

The Intercostal Muscles

The intercostals are the muscles involved with breathing that lie between the ribs. They are arranged as bands of muscle angling downward on the sides of the rib cage and the upper abdomen. They come into play by flexing the torso and causing it to twist. Performing any type of twisting crunch on a fitness ball will stimulate this group maximally.

The Serratus Muscles

The serratus anterior muscles are the finger–like strands of muscle on the rib cage, located between the front abs and the lats. Their job is to depress the rib cage as well as to assist in bringing the upper arms from a position pointing directly up from the shoulders to one pointing directly below the shoulders. A good exercise to stimulate these muscles is the one–arm cable crunch (using an overhead pulley).

EQUIPMENT NEEDED

Because this program focuses on building mass definition in your chest and arms, the workout routines primarily utilize dumbbell–based exercises as well as some machine exercises. There's been a lot of debate in recent years as to whether free weights are "better" than machines. Which one you use depends upon your goals, on your level of fitness, and on your likes. Here are some of the distinguishing characteristics of each method of training.

Free–weight exercises recruit the most muscle, so in order to get the fastest results, free–weights are preferable. Why? Your body is designed to be in a three–dimensional universe—we move in three planes: the sagittal (flexion and extension), transverse (internal and external rotation), and frontal (abduction and adduction). Free–weight training allows your body to move in a three–dimensional environment and involves not only training for a specific muscle group, but also balance, stability, and core training as well.

Whenever you use a machine, you limit your body to a two–dimensional universe and consequently you limit the number of muscle fibers that are going to do work. However machines often are safer and easier to use, especially for a newcomer to strength training. They are also fabulous if you have an injury and still want to work out. For example, you may have a strain in your lower back, which would make training your biceps in a standing position with dumbbells painful and unsafe. Instead, you can perform a curl using the biceps machine, or simply sit, alleviating additional strain to your lower back. Machines also are great for isolating certain hard to reach muscles and can be used to provide a different sort of tension to the working muscles, as in the example of a barbell curl versus a cable curl or an overhead dumbbell triceps extension versus an overhead cable extension.

In the end, as we always stress, variety is the spice of exercise. Mix them up; emphasize free weights, but supplement with some machines and other equipment, to keep your muscles and your mind constantly challenged in different ways.

We also include several exercises that utilize a fitness ball. As we mentioned before, you can purchase a ball at any sports store or online. These balls have grown tremendously in popularity during the last decade. They are great because they incorporate stability, posture, balance, and core training—thereby involving greater recruitment of muscle fibers. Small, firmer balls are more challenging than larger, soft balls. If you are de–conditioned you may want to start with a larger, soft ball until you've built up your core and stability strength. In general, the size ball you choose depends on your height: If you are 5′1″ to 5′7″ select a ball 55 cm in diameter; if you are 5′8″ to 6′2″ choose a 65 cm ball; if over 6′2″ use a 75″ ball.

SELECTING WEIGHT

The weight you select for each exercise depends on the number of repetitions that you need to do for a particular set. First, some definitions: A **rep,** or **repetition,** is when you perform an exercise (for example a bicep curl) one time. A **set** is made up of a given number of repetitions of the same exercise (for example a set of chest presses may consist of 12 presses).

In general, you want to keep your repetition range between 6 and 12 maximum. Research shows that the greatest strength and sculpting gains occur when you perform between 6 to 12 repetitions of an exercise with weight that is heavy enough that you feel like you cannot do another **repetition** with good form past the twelfth one. This is called the point of momentary **muscular failure**—weight training is one of the few activities in life where you succeed by failing!

HOW TO CHOOSE YOUR WEIGHT

Choosing the amount of weight needed for a particular exercise is simple. If you are told to do between 10 and 12 repetitions for one set, then you need to pick a weight where you fail (the point at which completing another repetition in good form becomes impossible) between 10 and 12 reps. This takes a bit of practice, but after a while you will become extremely accurate at choosing the correct weight for a particular repetition range. If you pick a weight that allows you to do more than 12 repetitions, you'll need to increase the amount of weight being lifted on the next set. If you reach failure before hitting the tenth rep, you'll need to decrease the amount of weight being lifted on the next set. When you get to the point where you can no longer lift a particular weight for a pre–determined repetition range, simply decrease the weight and prepare yourself for the next set. Conversely, when you fail to reach failure by the end of a repetition, it is time to increase the weight.

TRAINER'S NOTE: In the past people were told to determine their one–rep–maximum (which is the heaviest weight you can lift once and only once) and then work at 60 to 80 percent of that weight. This is dangerous for most people (especially beginners), since you may lift a weight that is way too heavy for your joints to handle while trying to determine your one-rep maximum. Instead of trying to find your one-rep max, we advise you to select your weights based on the number of repetitions prescribed by the parameters in the workout program.

LIFTING TECHNIQUES

PROPER BREATHING

The correct way to breathe while performing an exercise is to exhale (breathe out) while you are forcing the weight up (the concentric phase of the exercise or muscle contraction) and to inhale (breathe in) while you are lowering or releasing the weight (the eccentric phase or the negative portion of the exercise). For example, if you are doing a chest press, you exhale while you push the weight up away from your body and inhale while you lower the weight down toward your chest.

If you are lifting heavy weights, be careful that you don't inadvertently hold your breath. We have seen this technique used by many gym goers and it often leads to injury such as causing stroke due to increased blood pressure. The technical term for this is called a Valsalva maneuver, used mostly by power lifters. The Valsalva maneuver is performed by attempting to forcibly exhale while keeping the mouth and nose closed. This technique can be very dangerous and should be avoided at all costs.

SPEED OF LIFTING

While there has been interest recently in very slow lifting of weights, we have found that it is good only for beginners who are new to weight lifting. It helps them to learn and master the movement and prevents them from using bad exercise form. However, science, and our own experience, indicate that as you become more advanced, you should lift the weight as quickly as possible during the concentric portion without sacrificing form and without involving momentum (jerking and bouncing of the weights). You create more force by lifting faster and therefore more muscle fibers need to be activated.

If you do not use momentum to help move the weight, you can be sure that the force you generate during the movement is created solely by your muscles and not by momentum. This is what helps stimulate your muscles to grow, creating the tone and shape that you so desire.

While some believe that super–slow lifting is beneficial because it is difficult to perform and painful, it is not the best way to stimulate muscle growth. Super–slow lifting generates too much lactic acid within your muscles and fatigues them before they reach real momentary muscular failure.

Science tells us that Force = Mass (in this case the weight you are lifting) times Acceleration (the increasing speed at which you lift the weight). Therefore, the best way to lift weights is to lift them at a relatively fast rate (approximately two seconds to perform each rep on the way up) with total control of the weight and void of momentum. Then take three to four seconds on the way down. Since you won't be jerking the weights or using ballistic movements during exercise, the risk of getting injured is no greater than the risk of getting injured lifting super slowly.

A couple of last things about lifting speed:

1. The eccentric part of the movement, or the part where the weight is lowered (as in a barbell curl when you lower the bar to your thighs), needs to be performed in a slower, more controlled manner. Research indicates that the negative portion of the movement is of utmost importance for strength and mass gains. Also, an accelerated movement on the eccentric portion could lead to injury. Therefore, a controlled speed of three to four seconds is recommended.

2. If you are lifting a weight that allows you to do only 8 repetitions, it will look like you are lifting the weight slowly even though you are lifting it as fast as possible. This is due to the fact that the heavier weight is more difficult to move, even though you are trying to accelerate as fast as you can.

THE PROGRAM

The Chest & Arms Workout is a six–week program (except for the beginner phase), consisting of four upper body workouts each week, which focuses on the musculature of the Chest & Arms. There are three levels of workouts: beginner, intermediate, and advanced. Consider yourself a beginner if you are new to weight training or have been training for less than three months. Use the intermediate program if you have under a year of weight training and if your main goal is to gain definition and shape up the chest and arm area. If you have been training for a bit longer and would like to mainly increase muscle mass, then you can try the advanced program.

ZONE–TONE FOR MAXIMUM RESULTS

We are strong advocates of using a technique that we've developed—called the Zone–Tone method—to maximize your fitness gains. This method uses the mind–to–muscle connection, coupled with proper exercise technique and form, in order to most effectively stimulate your muscle fibers during an exercise. It involves really thinking about the muscles you are training right before you perform an exercise. In so doing, you increase mental focus and pre–isolate specific muscles.

When you effectively communicate with a specific muscle and prepare it for the upcoming set (work load), you have successfully engaged the mind–to–muscle connection. By keeping this connection active throughout the duration of the exercise, just one set can produce the results of five sets! Do you realize what this can do for you?! If you implement these principles in your training regimen, you will create unbelievably toned and incredibly defined muscles in half the time!

TO ZONE–TONE:

1. Zone in on the individual muscles you are training before each exercise. Concentrate on those muscles. Next, tense and contract (flex) those muscles as hard as you can before you actually begin the contraction. Here is where you engage and begin making the mind–to–muscle connection.

2. Maintain your mind–to–muscle connection during the execution of the exercise: Throughout the execution of the exercise, deliberately feel the muscle elongate (stretch) and contract (or flex), as you move along from point A to point B (the full range of movement for a particular exercise). What we really want you to do while you are performing the exercise is to contract (flex) the muscle as hard as you can in the same way that you did in step one, but

this time you'll have a weight in your hand, and add movement. This is crucial, as it is of no benefit to activate the muscles before the exercise if the mind–to–muscle connection is lost when the movement begins. Most people waste their time by exercising without thinking about what they're doing. They exercise on a physical plane rather than on both the mental and physical planes. This is fine if you are content with average results, but who really wants to be average? If you want to compound your results exponentially and create the body you've always dreamt about, you must effectively develop the mind–to–muscle connection.

HOW TO FURTHER ENHANCE ZONE–TONE'S EFFECT?

How would you like to multiply the effects of the Zone–Tone method? Here is a way to compound your results with little or no additional time expenditure.

When you're getting ready for bed at night, before you get too sleepy, practice the following protocol: Start with your feet as you begin to relax and focus upon your toes, slightly wiggling them and concentrating on feeling even the slightest movement in each individual toe. You might actually feel a little strange tingling sensation because you have never before paid attention to the feeling of these individual parts of your body. You might wonder why we would waste time focusing on the feet first. We want you to become completely familiar and in sync with each and every part of your body. This eventually will give you the ability to effectively isolate any muscle you desire. It is very important to remember to focus upon each and every part of your body, from the tips of your toes to the top of your head! As you move on from the feet toward your knees and up, zone in on every body part along the way.

KNOW YOUR GOALS

Without goals you are like a ship on the middle of the sea, just drifting away with no sense of direction. In order to achieve success we need to clearly define and ingrain our goals in our minds. Otherwise, like the drifting boat, if you get anywhere it will be by mere chance. Here are some tips for successful goal setting.

- **WRITE DOWN YOUR GOALS.** If they are in writing they will be clear and you can always return to them when you need reinforcement.

- **BE SPECIFIC.** What measurements do you want to have; what about your body fat percentage, and total body weight; how much larger do you want your muscles to be?

- **MAKE GOALS REALISTIC AND ATTAINABLE WITHIN THE TIMEFRAME.** If you have a body type for which muscle building is difficult, going from 16" to 20" biceps in four weeks is unrealistic. Know your body. Set yourself up for success, not failure.

For the next six weeks I will:

Lose	_____	pounds of fat
Gain	_____	pounds of muscle
Weigh	_____	pounds

Have measurements of:

Chest	_____	inches
Arms	_____	inches
Waist	_____	inches

Here's where it can get tricky. Simply focusing on the individual muscles of the body is not enough. When you simply think about them you cannot truly get a feel for how they feel as when they are in motion. To help you home in and actually gain a feel for each of these muscles, do the following:

- As you get to each individual body part, stop and contract the muscle as well as you know how. Do this three to five times and then relax. Hold each contraction for about 3 to 5 seconds and then relax for 5 seconds before you begin the next cycle.

- Remember the exact area where you felt the intended muscle contract and now focus all of your attention and energy on relaxing that same area. If you do this, you will aquire the ability to be in complete control of your entire superficial muscular system and will have the opportunity to call upon its action for maximum muscular efficiency.

Here is yet another technique you should use to further enhance the overall effects of the Zone–Tone method:

After you complete each set of an exercise, stand in the mirror and contract (flex) the muscles that you were exercising as hard as you can and hold for a count of 3 to 5 seconds. This will help you to create a stronger mind–to–muscle connection and to accurately identify and call upon those individual muscles during an exercise. In addition, it will help to bring more blood and nutrients to the intended muscle, for enhanced results.

We can't emphasize enough how important it is to practice the Zone–Tone method both when you're working out and while at rest. As with anything, the more you practice the Zone–Tone method the quicker you'll be able to do it, and the more powerful it will become. Soon you will realize, first hand, the astonishing results gained from this powerful concept. Good luck, train hard, and get in the zone!

The three workouts in the Chest & Arms Workout use the program technique known as periodization, which involves varying your strength–training program in fourteen–day intervals in order to prevent your body from adapting. In order for your muscles to continue to be challenged and for your body to keep realizing benefits, it needs to be surprised a bit—otherwise, you will find yourself at a plateau point where you are no longer getting leaner, or more sculpted. There are many ways that a program can be varied, as we have previously discussed—for example, you can change the types and order of exercises, the number of repetitions and sets you perform for each exercise, the speed of lifting, and the amount of rest time between exercises.

Periodization varies these variables in a logical and orderly manner in order to deliver the fastest results possible. Studies consistently show that people who train using the periodization approach realize greater gains than those whose routines remain the same.

Tied closely to the periodization concept is the principle of progression. In order for you to make any muscular gains, and to change the appearance of a muscle, you need to progress—that is constantly present your muscles with a challenge. Progression means increasing the weight that you lift, or the number of repetitions, or the number of sets that you do in order to increase the overall load on your body. To be effective and safe, slow and rational progress is critical. Do not suddenly increase your weight load by a great amount of weight. Test it out. See how heavy you can go and still perform the desired number of reps where you reach failure by the time you reach the end of a set.

Progression can also lead to an increased use of dumbbells and less reliance on machines as your balance and kinesthetic awareness improve, and as you gain enough strength to perform a free–weight exercise in good form.

You will find that the workouts in this book are different on each day of a given week, and that every two weeks, the workout changes in other, bigger ways, which include the number of reps/sets you perform and the amount of rest time in between exercises. The way it changes depends on whether you are doing the beginner, intermediate, or advanced version. For some two–week segments you might be performing **modified compound supersets**—performing back–to–back exercises for opposing muscle groups (for example your back and chest) or performing multiple exercises for the same muscle group (for example following a chest press with a fly) with the prescribed rest period in between each set.

For the following two–week periods you might switch to **supersetting**—you perform two exercises back–to–back without any rest in between. Finally, the biggest challenge comes from performing **giant sets**—four exercises performed one after the other with no rest between each exercise. The only rest time occurs at the end of the fourth set, before you cycle back to the first exercise. All three Chest & Arms Workouts also include abdominal and cardiovascular components.

HOW TO INCORPORATE CHEST & ARMS INTO THE BODY SCULPTING BIBLE WORKOUTS

There are several ways you can use the workouts presented in this book. If you are already following the 14–Day Body Sculpting Program from the original *Body Sculpting Bible for Men*, then just substitute the upper body workouts for the workouts presented in Part III of this book, once you finish the 6–week Body Sculpting Cycle of the original workout. Note; that the shoulder workout in the original books is performed with the leg workout, so you will need to eliminate the shoulder work from your leg day. Please refer to Part III of this book for more detail as to how to incorporate the workouts in your existing Body Sculpting Bible Program.

If this is the first book that you purchase from the *Body Sculpting Bible* series, please make sure that you incorporate two leg workouts per week so that you do not create an imbalanced physique. On Part III of the book, we also offer suggestions on when to include these workouts.

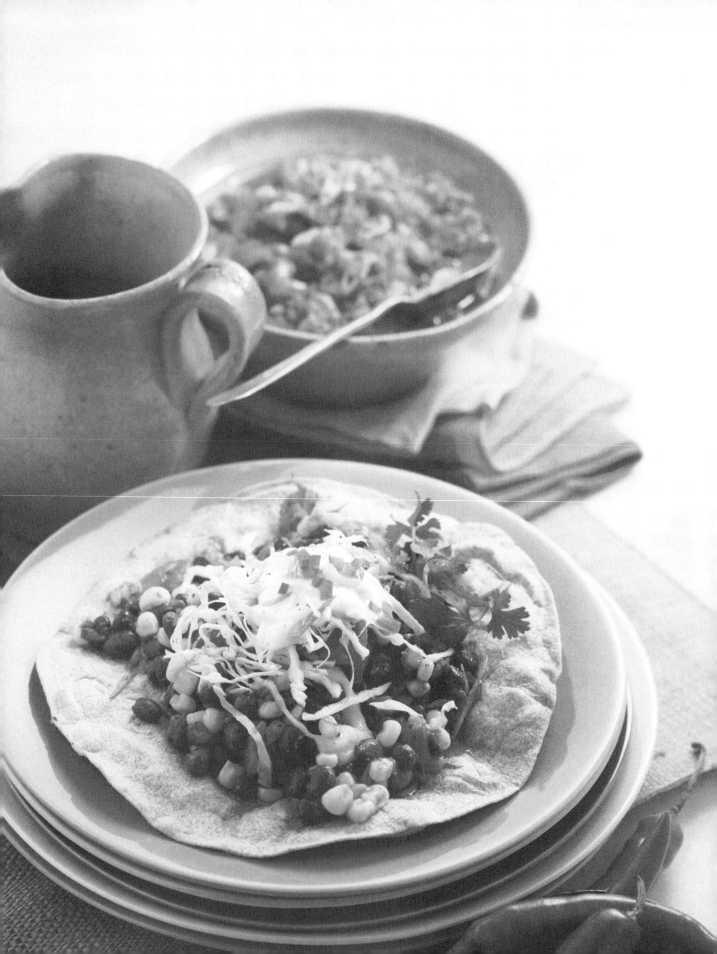

Chapter 2
Fitness Fuel

Working out and eating properly are both necessary to transform your upper body into a strong and, sculpted work of art. Even though you may think that working out gives you a license to eat whatever you want, whenever you want, it doesn't. Even the most rigorous exercise regimen will be undone by poor eating habits.

The nutritional approach that we find most effective for most healthy people is based on a principle of balance among the major nutrients that your body requires. However, some people—diabetics, for example—may have unique needs, so it is wise to check with a nutritionist or your doctor before radically changing your eating habits.

That said, the following guide-

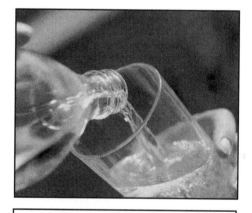

THE BODY SCULPTING BIBLE FOR CHEST & ARMS

2

lines and information will help you to formulate a diet that is rich in energy–producing nutrients—foods that provide the fuel you need to support and enhance your Chest & Arms Workout.

NECESSARY NUTRIENTS

There are three macronutrients that the human body needs in order to function properly: carbohydrates, proteins, and fats.

CARBOHYDRATES

Carbohydrates are your body's main source of energy. When you ingest carbohydrates, your pancreas releases a hormone called insulin. Insulin is very important because:

- It grabs the carbohydrates and either stores them in the muscle or stores them as fat.
- It grabs the amino acids (protein) and shelters them inside the muscle cell to be used for recovery and repair.

Most overweight people on low fat/high carbohydrate diets eat an overabundance of carbohydrates. Too many carbohydrates cause a huge release of insulin. When there is too much insulin in the body, your body turns into a fat–storing machine. Therefore, it is important to eat the right amount and kinds of carbohydrates.

Carbohydrates are divided into complex carbohydrates and simple carbohydrates. The complex carbohydrates give you sustained energy ("timed release") while the simple carbohydrates gives you immediate energy. It is recommended that you eat mainly complex carbohydrates throughout the day—except after your workout when your body needs simple carbohydrates in order to replenish its glycogen levels immediately, to help muscles recover and rebuild quickly.

There are two types of **complex carbohydrates:** starchy, such as those found in oatmeal, sweet potatoes, and grits; and fibrous, which are plentiful in broccoli, cauliflower, and zucchini. Examples of simple carbohydrates that are healthy include many fruits: apples, bananas, grapes, and oranges.

PROTEIN

Every tissue in your body is made from protein (i.e., muscle, hair, skin, and nails). Proteins are the building blocks of muscle tissue. Every time you eat protein your metabolism increases by approximately 20 percent, because the body needs to work hard to break down the complex protein molecules. In addition, protein enables carbohydrates to be time released, providing you with sustained energy throughout the day.

In a weight–training program such as the Chest & Arms Workout, you should consume between 1 gram to 1.5 grams of protein per pound of lean body mass (meaning that if you are 200 lbs, and have 10% body fat, you should consume no less than 180 g of protein and no more than 270 g, since your lean body mass = 180 lbs.). Consuming more than 1.5 grams of protein per pound of lean body mass is not recommended, as the body begins to metabolize the protein into glucose burned for energy. Also, there is no further muscle-building benefit from a higher protein intake.

Good examples of protein are eggs, chicken breast (cooked, skinless and boneless: 6 oz), turkey (cooked, skinless and boneless: 6 oz), lean (90% lean) red meats (6 oz), and tuna (6 oz).

Each serving size equals approximately 35 to 40 grams of protein.

FATS

There are three types of fats: saturated, polyunsaturated, and monounsaturated.

Saturated fats are associated with heart disease and high cholesterol levels. They are found to a large extent in products of animal origin. However, some vegetable fats are altered in a way that increases the amount of saturated fats in them by a chemical process known as hydrogenation. Hydrogenated vegetable oils are generally found in packaged foods; these oils should be avoided at all costs as they have been shown to play a huge role in causing insulin resistance, clogged arteries, and obesity. In addition, coconut oil, palm oil, and palm kernel oil, which are also frequently used in packaged foods, and non–dairy creamers, are also highly saturated.

Polyunsaturated fats do not have an effect in cholesterol levels. Most of the fats in vegetable oils, such as canola oil, corn oil, cottonseed, safflower, soybean, and sunflower oil are polyunsaturated. Flaxseed oil and fish oils are also polyunsaturated. These last two should be the main source of your polyunsaturated fat consumption. If you use flaxseed oil make sure

that it is bottled in a dark container that protects it from light. Keep it refrigerated because heat makes it rancid (therefore never cook with it). These last two fats are usually high in the Omega-3 essential fatty acids and may have antioxidant properties. Corn oil, on the other hand should never be used for cooking as it contributes to increases in the size of fat cells.

Monounsaturated fats have a health–enhancing effect because they lower the levels of LDL (bad cholesterol) and increase the levels of HDL (good cholesterol). Sources of these fats are extra virgin olive oil and nuts such as cashews, pecans and almonds. Peanut butter fits in here too but the peanut is really a bean rather than a nut. The main source of your monounsaturated fats should be canned extra virgin olive oil.

We recommend that 20 percent of your calories come from good fats. Any less than 20% and your hormonal production decreases. Any more than 20% and you start accumulating plenty of fat. Good sources of fat are extra virgin olive oil from a can (1 tablespoon), natural peanut butter (2 tablespoons), flaxseed oil (1 tablespoon), and fish oils (1 tablespoon). Each serving size contains approximately 12 to 16 grams of fat.

In our approach to nutrition, we use a diet that contains all of the macronutrients in a more balanced manner. The breakdown of the nutrients looks like this:

40% Carbs
40% Protein
20% Fats

CHARACTERISTICS OF A GOOD NUTRITION PROGRAM

- **Your nutrition plan should be based on eating small and frequent meals throughout the day.** Aim for eating five or six small meals each day, with two to three hours between each meal, rather than a couple of large ones.

- **All meals should contain carbohydrates, protein, and fat in the correct ratios.** Balancing each meal ensures that your body is fueled with energy in the proper proportion to maximize power.

- **Do not smoke, and limit alcohol consumption.** Both lower testosterone levels (in addition to presenting many other potential health problems). Alcohol in particular is responsible for increased fat gain: each gram of alcohol has 7 calories. To make matters worse, alcohol not only increases your blood sugar levels, which in turn signals the body to produce insulin (remember that too much insulin prevents fat from being burned), but also, once your blood sugar goes down again, your appetite will go up. Not good when you are trying to get in shape.

- **Hydrate Frequently.** Nearly 65 percent of our bodies are composed of water. It is always important to make sure you drink enough, especially if you are working out. A good rule of thumb is to multiply your body weight by 0.66 in ounces of water per day. For instance, if you weigh 200 lbs, then you need to consume 132 ounces of water per day.

CALORIC NEEDS

Caloric requirements for most men fluctuate between 2,000 and 2,500 calories per day. However, if you eat the same number of calories day in and day out your body will adapt to that number of calories and you will stop losing fat. To prevent this, we recommend that you alternate between consuming 2,000 and 2,500 calories every two weeks.

Once you know the total number of calories you need to take in every day, calculate the amount (in grams) of each nutrient by using the percentages above:

Total amount of carbs for the day = (Total number of calories x 0.40)/4

Total amount of protein for the day = (Total number of calories x 0.40)/4

Total amount of fat for the day = (Total number of calories x 0.20)/9

Note: Carbs and protein are divided by 4 because there are 4 calories per gram of carbs or of protein. For fats, we divide by 9 since there are 9 calories for every gram of fat).

Divide all of the results from the formulas above by five (or by six, if you are eating six times a day), to obtain the amount of each nutrient that you will need to consume at each meal.

2,000-CALORIE WEEKS MACRONUTRIENT REQUIREMENTS

200 grams of carbohydrates (mostly complex, with simple carbs being saved for after the workout)

200 grams of protein

45 grams of fats

In five meals that comes out to approximately:

40 grams of carbs per meal

40 grams of protein per meal

9 grams of fats per meal

The next section features a chart indicating what specific foods to eat at each meal.

CHOOSING FOOD

One of the biggest challenges that we face when starting a diet is deciding what to eat every day. Now that you have calculated the amount of carbs, protein and fats you need for each meal, you need to choose what foods to eat. For this purpose the food–groups table found on the next page contains the food values for the foods we recommend you eat. It is very accurate. However, if you happen to discover a discrepancy between the nutritional information on a food label and the chart, use the information from the food label.

The following chart indicates the types and quantities of foods to choose for each one of your meals. The times are, of course, approximate and you can change them based on your own schedule. For the post–workout meal, we assume that you are training in the morning, but if this is not the case, have some complex carbs in the morning and move the post–workout meal to after your workout.

2,500-CALORIE WEEK MACRONUTRIENT REQUIREMENTS

250 grams of carbohydrates (mostly complex, with simple carbs being saved for after the workout)

250 grams of protein

55 grams of fats

In six meals that comes out to approximately:

42 grams of carbs per meal

42 grams of protein per meal

9 grams of fats per meal

2,000-CALORIE WEEKS

MEAL 1 (7:30 AM)–BREAKFAST
CHOOSE 40 GRAMS FROM GROUP A
CHOOSE 40 GRAMS FROM GROUP C

MEAL 2 (10:30 AM)–MORNING BREAK SNACK
CHOOSE 40 GRAMS FROM GROUP A
CHOOSE 40 GRAMS FROM GROUP B

MEAL 3 (1:30 PM)–LUNCH TIME
CHOOSE 40 GRAMS FROM GROUP A
CHOOSE 30 GRAMS FROM GROUP B
CHOOSE 10 GRAMS FROM GROUP D

MEAL 4 (3:30 PM)–AFTERNOON BREAK SNACK
CHOOSE 40 GRAMS FROM GROUP A
CHOOSE 40 GRAMS FROM GROUP B

MEAL 5 (6:30 PM)–DINNER
CHOOSE 40 GRAMS FROM GROUP A
CHOOSE 25 GRAMS FROM GROUP B
CHOOSE 15 GRAMS FROM GROUP D

2,500-CALORIE WEEKS

MEAL 1 (7:30 AM)–BREAKFAST
CHOOSE 42 GRAMS FROM GROUP A
CHOOSE 42 GRAMS FROM GROUP C

MEAL 2 (10:30 AM)–MORNING BREAK SNACK
CHOOSE 42 GRAMS FROM GROUP A
CHOOSE 42 GRAMS FROM GROUP B

MEAL 3 (1:30 PM)–LUNCH TIME
CHOOSE 42 GRAMS FROM GROUP A
CHOOSE 12 GRAMS FROM GROUP B
CHOOSE 10 GRAMS FROM GROUP D

MEAL 4 (3:30 PM)–AFTERNOON BREAK SNACK
CHOOSE 42 GRAMS FROM GROUP A
CHOOSE 42 GRAMS FROM GROUP B

MEAL 5 (6:30 PM)–EARLY DINNER
CHOOSE 42 GRAMS FROM GROUP A
CHOOSE 27 GRAMS FROM GROUP B
CHOOSE 15 GRAMS FROM GROUP D

MEAL 6 (8:30 PM)–LATE DINNER
CHOOSE 42 GRAMS FROM GROUP A
CHOOSE 22 GRAMS FROM GROUP B
CHOOSE 20 GRAMS FROM GROUP D

Note: Include 1 tsp of olive oil three times a day with any meals (except the post workout meal) on one day. The next day, include one tsp of olive oil once a day and one tsp of flax seed oil twice a day with any meals (except the post–workout meal). This, in conjunction with the naturally occurring fats in the food, will cover your essential fats needs.

Note: Include 1 tsp of olive oil three times a day with any meals (except the post–workout meal) on one day. The next day, include one tsp of olive oil once a day and one tsp of flax oil twice a day with any meals (except the post workout meal). This, in conjunction with the naturally occurring fats in the food, will cover your essential fats needs.

FOOD GROUP TABLES

For the post–workout meal (meal that comes after the workout is performed), choose 1 item from Group A and 1 item from Group C in order to create a balanced meal. For all other meals, choose 1 item from Group A, 1 item from Group B, and 1 item from Group D in order to create a balanced meal. Remember to adjust the serving size depending upon the amount of nutrients that you require per meal.

GROUP A – PROTEINS

FOOD	GRAMS	FOOD	GRAMS
Chicken breast (3.5 oz. broiled)	35	WhiteFish (3.5 oz broiled)	31
Tuna fish (spring water) 3.5 oz	35	Halibut (3.5 oz broiled)	31
Turkey breast (3.5 oz broiled)	28	Cod (3.5 oz broiled)	31
Whey protein (2 scoops)	20	Round steak (3.5 oz Broiled)	33

GROUP B – COMPLEX CARBOHYDRATES

FOOD	GRAMS	FOOD	GRAMS
Baked potato (3.5 oz)	21	Rice (white or brown) (2/3 cup)	31
Plain oatmeal (1/2 cup dry)	27	Shredded wheat (1 cup dry)	31
Plain pasta (1 cup)	44	Corn (1/2 cup)	31
Whole-wheat bread (1 slice)	12	Yams (3 oz baked or roasted)	21

GROUP C – SIMPLE CARBOHYDRATES

FOOD	GRAMS	FOOD	GRAMS
Apple (1 fruit)	15	Banana (6 oz)	27
Cantaloupe (1 fruit)	25	Grapes (1 cup)	14
Strawberries (1 cup)	9	Yogurt (1 serving)	27

GROUP D – FIBROUS CARBOHYDRATES

FOOD (10 OZ SERVING)	GRAMS	FOOD (10 OZ SERVING)	GRAMS
Asparagus	25	Squash	25
Broccoli	25	Green Beans	25
Cabbage	25	Cauliflower	25
Celery	25	Cucumber	25
Mushrooms	25	Lettuce	25
Red or Green Peppers	25	Tomato	25
Spinach	25	Zucchini	25

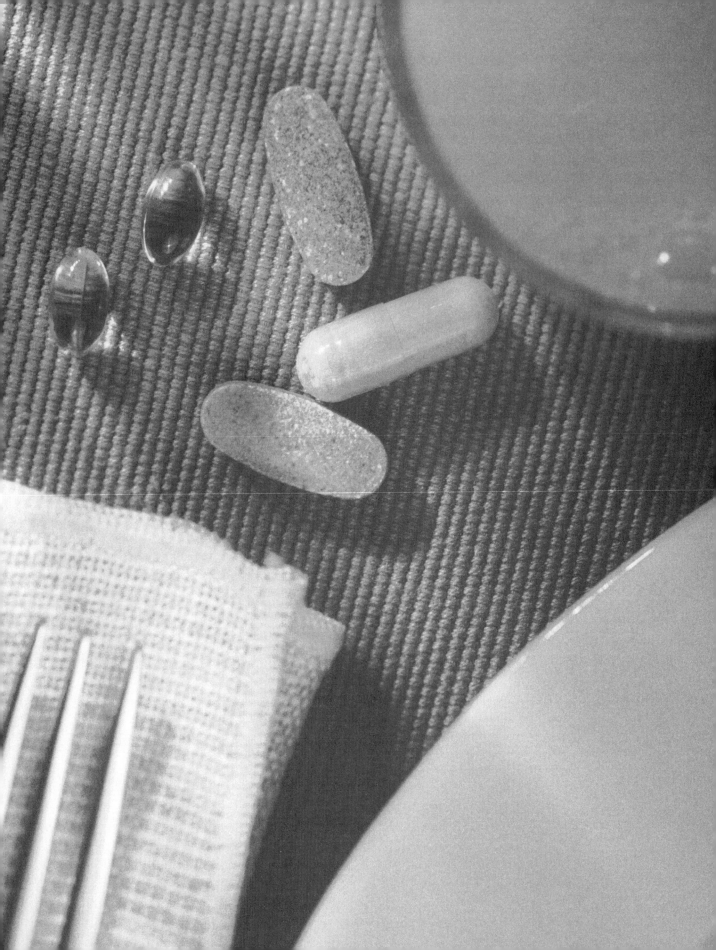

SHOULD YOU SUPPLEMENT?

Because today's foods are so processed, it is impossible to get all of the nutrients that the body needs to function properly from food alone. Because of this, it is necessary to use nutritional supplements to insure that our bodies have everything they need for repair and growth. Here are our recommendations:

- A good **multiple vitamin and mineral formula** taken preferably with your post–workout meal or at breakfast on non–workout days in order to avoid any nutritional deficiencies.

- **Chromium picolinate** (200 mcg) also with the post–workout meal or at breakfast. This mineral is good for increasing the cells' acceptance of the hormone insulin. Good insulin sensitivity is necessary in order to optimize the fat burning process. **Note:** Some multiple vitamin/mineral formulas already contain this mineral, so check the label.

- 1000 mg of **vitamin C** three times a day. Start with only 500 mg and increase the dosage by 500 mg per week until you reach the 3000 mg total. (This will prevent stomach problems.) Vitamin C is thought to reduce levels of cortisol , the stress hormone released by the adrenal glands that likes to eat muscle and store fat.

- **Whey protein shakes or meal replacement shakes like Prolab's Lean Mass Complex,** or any other similar formula, are useful while you are on the go and cannot have a real meal. We recommend Prolab's Lean Mass Complex because it is based on complex carbohydrates and a blend of different proteins consisting of a 40/40/20 macronutrient ratio. It contains 40 grams of carbs, 40 grams of proteins and 8 grams of fats, making it the perfect meal replacement supplement for this program. The product is also easy to prepare; it requires no blender—just some water and a spoon and the taste is fantastic.

Part 2
The Exercises

It's time to introduce the exercises that comprise your Chest & Arms Workout. We begin with a chapter on stretching to improve flexibility, and continue with muscle-building exercises for your chest, back and shoulders, and biceps and triceps. Carefully read the description of each exercise, making recommended modifications to fit your fitness level and goals.

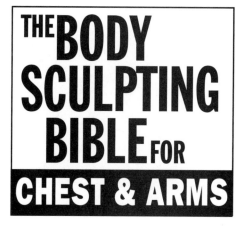

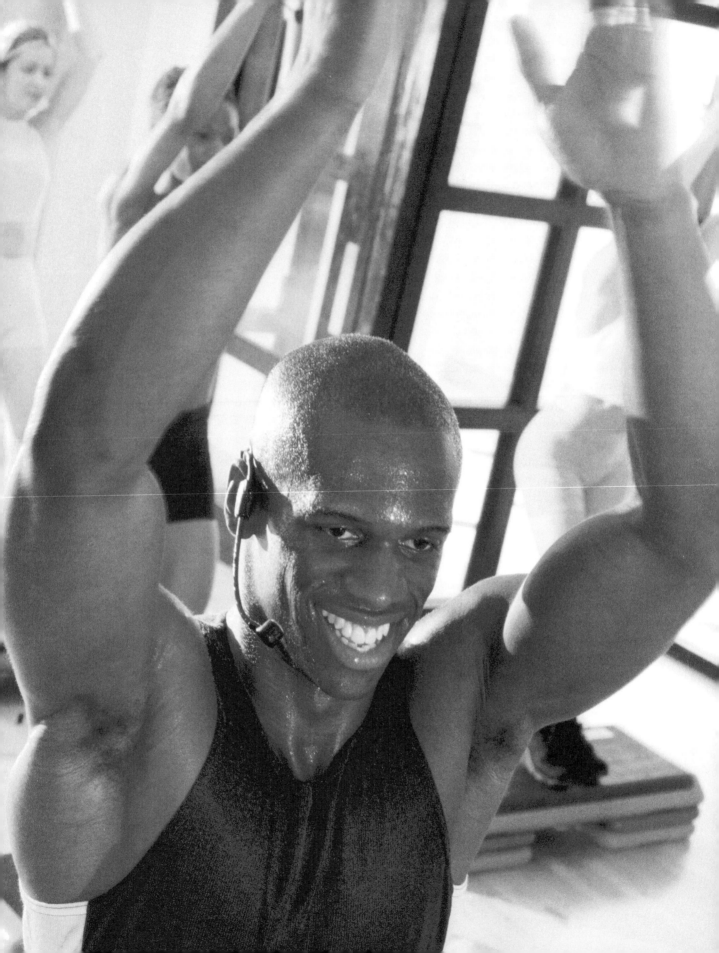

Chapter 3

Many of our clients don't like to take the time to stretch out their muscles. We understand. If you are pressed for time, it is easy to forgo the stretch component of your workout because you feel that it's not doing much of anything. But in fact, the pre–workout warm up and post–workout stretch are vital components of your Chest & Arms Workout. And they don't require a lot of time—just a few minutes. The next few pages will show you how to warm up most effectively for your workout and how to stretch out your muscles to prevent injury.

ACTIVELY WARM UP BEFORE YOU BEGIN

Research indicates that you should perform an active warm up before you begin a workout. The key word here is active. In the past, people were told to perform holding stretches (called static stretches) before they worked out—for example, stretching your legs before going for a run. However, the most recent research, including one major review of the research on stretching conducted by researchers at SMBD–Jewish General Hospital in Montreal,

Ultimate Stretching

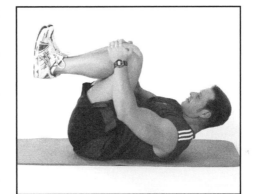

THE BODY SCULPTING BIBLE FOR CHEST & ARMS

3

has found that stretching before you exercise does not prevent injury. In certain cases, if you stretch right before an activity you actually increase your risk for injury because the stretch can temporarily reduce force and power in your muscle. Instead, it is recommended that you stretch after your workout to improve your range of motion on a regular basis, a few times a week.

Before you work out, you want to increase your heart rate and prepare your body for the work ahead. This is best achieved through an active warm up, which increases blood flow to your muscles, preparing your neuromuscular system for the movements you will need to perform.

The best active warm-up for the Chest & Arms Workout consists of about five minutes of movement involving large muscles in your body. For example, a combination of squats (body weight only), jumping jacks, jogging or fast walking, or five minutes on a elliptical trainer that includes a rowing motion for your arms. In your warm up you want to try to use all of the upper body muscles you will be working during workout.

It is also very helpful to warm up by emulating some of the actual weight-lifting exercises you will perform during your workout. For example, if your workout is to consist of biceps curls and triceps kickbacks, your warm up could include performing those exercises with little or no weight. This is an effective way to prepare your body and mind for the workout by increasing your kinesthetic awareness and by moving blood to the muscles that will be working. It also enhances safety by providing an opportunity to practice proper form before you perform the exercise with resistance.

STATIC STRETCH AT THE END, NOT BEGINNING OF YOUR WORKOUT

While there's scant evidence that static stretching (the type of stretch that involves holding a stretched position for a number of seconds with no bouncing) before your workout prevents injury, you can do a few pre-workout stretches that are dynamic. Dynamic stretches involve performing several repetitions of bringing a muscle quickly into a stretched position and then immediately releasing it. This type of stretching helps to prepare your muscles for the workout ahead.

The optimal, safest time to do static stretching is at the end of the workout. This is when your muscles are warm due to increased blood flow that occurred during your workout. Therefore, it is the best time to elongate them. In addition, there's less risk of causing injury by overstretching when the muscles are warm. In contrast, if you perform static stretches on cold muscles (for example, first thing in the morning), your range of motion is much more limited and you risk pushing the stretch too far and injuring the muscle or connective tissues.

There are two ways you can perform the static stretches in the Chest & Arms Workout. You may opt to perform a stretch for a particular muscle group during your rest period right after you have completed all the sets of exercises for that group (for example, your chest) and before you move on to the next set of exercises. Or, you may perform all of the static stretches at the very end of your workout.

THE PROPER WAY TO STRETCH

The way you stretch makes all the difference between an effective, fitness–enhancing stretch and a dangerous one. First, begin your static stretch by inhaling from your diaphragm (the base of your lungs) rather than from your chest (a helpful mental image is to imagine you are inflating a balloon with your breathing). As you move into the stretch position, exhale. Go deep enough into a stretch to feel tension in the muscles you are stretching. Never force a stretch. Hold the stretch position for 10 to 30 seconds before releasing. Continue to breathe deeply while in the stretch position. Never hold your breath.

As you hold the stretch, you will begin to feel your muscles moving from a state of tension to relaxation. At this point, you can try to take the stretch a bit deeper. It is normal to feel some discomfort during the initial moments of the stress; if you feel any pain, however, ease up on the stretch immediately. During a static stretch you want to hold the stretch without any bouncing (ballistic stretching). While ballistic stretching has its place in preparing the body for some athletic moves, it is not recommended at the end of your Chest & Arms Workout program.

UPPER BODY STRETCH PROGRAM

The stretches that appear on the following pages can be done dynamically before your workout, or statically afterward. Before your workout, perform several repetitions of each stretch, holding each one for only 1 to 3 seconds. (Also, remember you can simulate the

---

BEYOND STATIC

While the stretch program for the Chest & Arms Workout is static in nature, you may want to know about a couple of other effective stretching techniques.

- **PNF:** Short for proprioceptive neuromuscular facilitation, this type of stretching quickens the response of your neuromuscular system. To perform a PNF stretch, first perform a five– to ten–second isometric contraction of a muscle (tense the muscle without moving it) and then release the tension, while someone else presses you further into the stretch. PNF stretches increase your mobility as they allow you to take a stretch deeper than is possible with static stretching. This stretch is to be performed by advanced atheletes only under the supervision of very experienced fitness trainers.

- **AI–STRETCH:** Active–isolated stretches involve active flexibility exercises to isolate the muscle you want to stretch. The principle behind A–I stretch is to fire up or contract the primary muscle (agonist) to place the opposing muscle (antagonist) in a state of relaxation. (Whenever you contract a muscle, its opposite muscle relaxes or stretches). For example, if you want to do an A–I stretch for your biceps you actively contract your triceps (the opposing muscle group) by performing a kickback extension. Then, using a towel or assistant, add intensity, and hold the stretch for $1\frac{1}{2}$ to 2 seconds before releasing repeating it. These stretches are usually done 8 to 12 times per muscle.

---

actual exercises you will do in your workout for your warm up). After your workout, perform one repetition of each stretch but hold without bouncing for as long as 30 seconds.

NECK STRETCH

During upper–body workout exercises, people often lift their shoulders and place strain on their necks while trying to execute a movement. Perform this stretch at the beginning of your stretch routine to relieve any tension you may be holding in your neck.

TECHNIQUE AND FORM

❶ Start in a standing position.

❷ With your hand on your head, press your head over to your right shoulder. Hold for a few seconds. Release.

❸ Press your head toward your left shoulder. Hold for a few seconds. Release.

❹ Press your head down toward your chest. Hold for a few seconds. Release.

TRAINER'S TIPS

✖ Make sure you are not applying too much pressure to your head. You want to feel a tension in your neck, without any pain. Don't forget to breathe throughout the stretch.

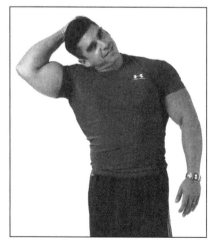
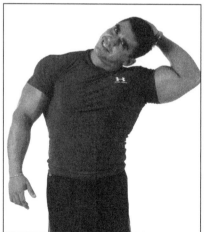
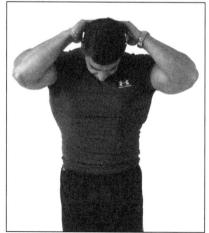

UPPER BACK AND BICEPS STRETCH

This terrific stretch is for the muscles in the mid- and upper back, and the fronts of your arms.

TECHNIQUE AND FORM

1 Start in a standing position.

2 Interlock your fingers and exhale as you press your arms forward (palms facing front); pull your abs into your spine, and round your chest.

3 Hold for 10 to 30 seconds.

TRAINER'S TIPS

⊗ Keep your knees slightly bent as you perform the stretch.

⊗ Your legs should remain still while you stretch—only your arms and torso move.

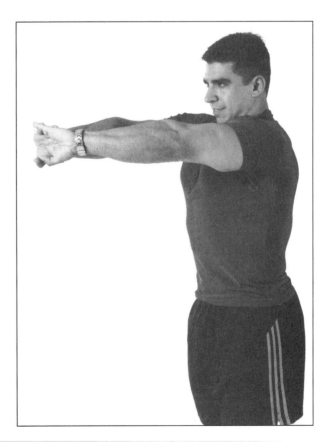

WALL CHEST STRETCH

This stretch opens the muscles in your chest, improving your posture and preventing injury.

TECHNIQUE AND FORM

1 Stand facing a wall, with your right arm extended and hand pressed against the wall.

2 Lean into the wall and then twist your torso away from it, until you feel the stretch in the right side of your chest and upper arm.

3 Hold for 10 to 30 seconds.

TRAINER'S TIPS

✖ If your shoulder hurts, release the stretch immediately.

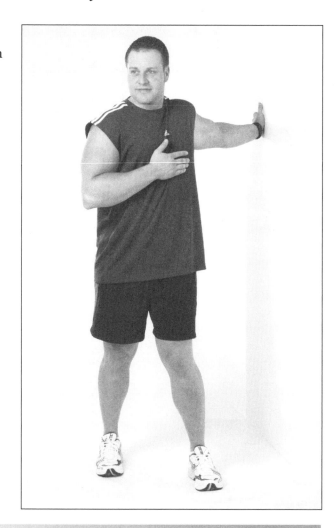

EXTENDED ARMS CHEST STRETCH

This simple stretch can be done anytime, anywhere to release muscular tension in the chest and the shoulders.

TECHNIQUE AND FORM

1 Start in standing position.

2 Bring your arms behind your back and interlock your fingers.

3 Extend your chest forward as you lift your arms while simultaneously pressing through your palms.

TRAINER'S TIPS

Try not to overarch your back (a bit of arching is natural).

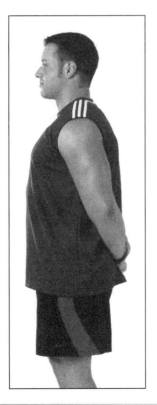
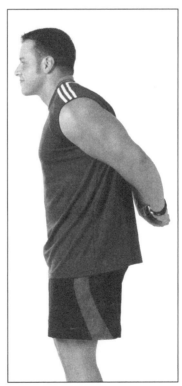

TRICEPS STRETCH

When you perform the triceps stretch for the backs of your arms, make sure that you concentrate on reaching your hand down your back as you press your elbow in.

TECHNIQUE AND FORM

1 Stand or sit cross–legged.

2 Reach your right arm straight overhead, then bend it so that your right hand is reaching down your back.

3 Use your left hand to press your right elbow close to your head; at the same time reach down your back with your right hand.

4 Hold for 10 to 30 seconds and then perform the same stretch with other arm.

TRAINER'S TIPS

✪ Exhale deeply as you reach your hand down your back.

✪ Make sure your fingers remain unclenched.

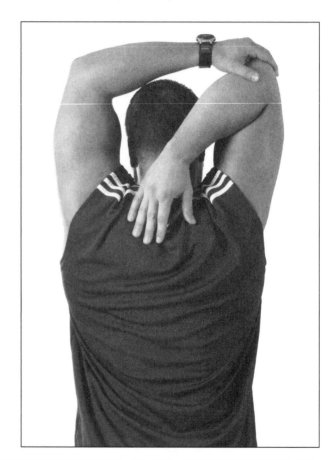

SHOULDER STRETCH

Make sure you keep your shoulder down as you perform this stretch.

TECHNIQUE AND FORM

1 Stand straight. Grasp one of your elbows with the opposite hand.

1 Without moving your torso, pull your arm as far as possible toward your body.

1 Hold for 10 to 30 seconds before repeating with other arm.

TRAINER'S TIPS

Keep your arm parallel to the floor as you pull it toward your body.

Keep your legs about shoulder width apart for balance and support.

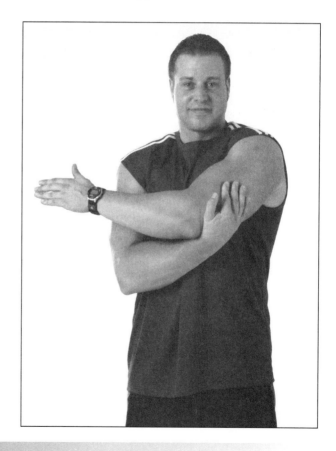

LYING LOWER BACK STRETCH

This relaxing stretch releases the tension in your lower back and is easy to do.

TECHNIQUE AND FORM

1 Begin lying on your back (supine position), with your legs extended in front of you and your arms by your sides.

2 Exhale as you bend your knees and hug them tightly, bringing them toward your chest.

3 Hold for 10 to 30 seconds.

TRAINER'S TIPS

Concentrate on pressing your knees in, breathe deeply, and you'll feel an immediate release of pressure in your spine. Keep your shoulders on the floor throughout the stretch.

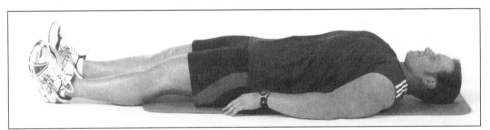

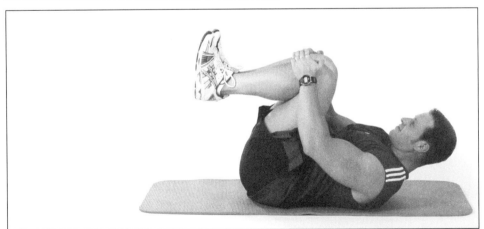

BACK STRETCH ON THE BALL

This stretch really feels great all along your entire vertebral column. Ease into it and enjoy.

TECHNIQUE AND FORM

1 Begin sitting on the ball; slide down so that your back is on the ball.

2 Roll your body back until it arches over the ball. Your head will be on one side of the ball, your feet on the other.

3 Hold for 10 to 30 seconds, then walk your legs forward to return to a seated position.

TRAINER'S TIPS

Keep your head back, so that you release tension from your cervical vertebrae through your lumbar spine.

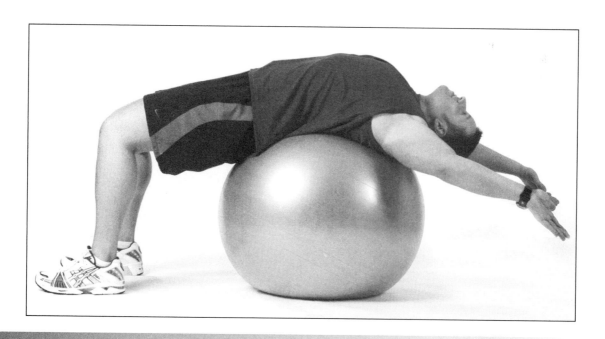

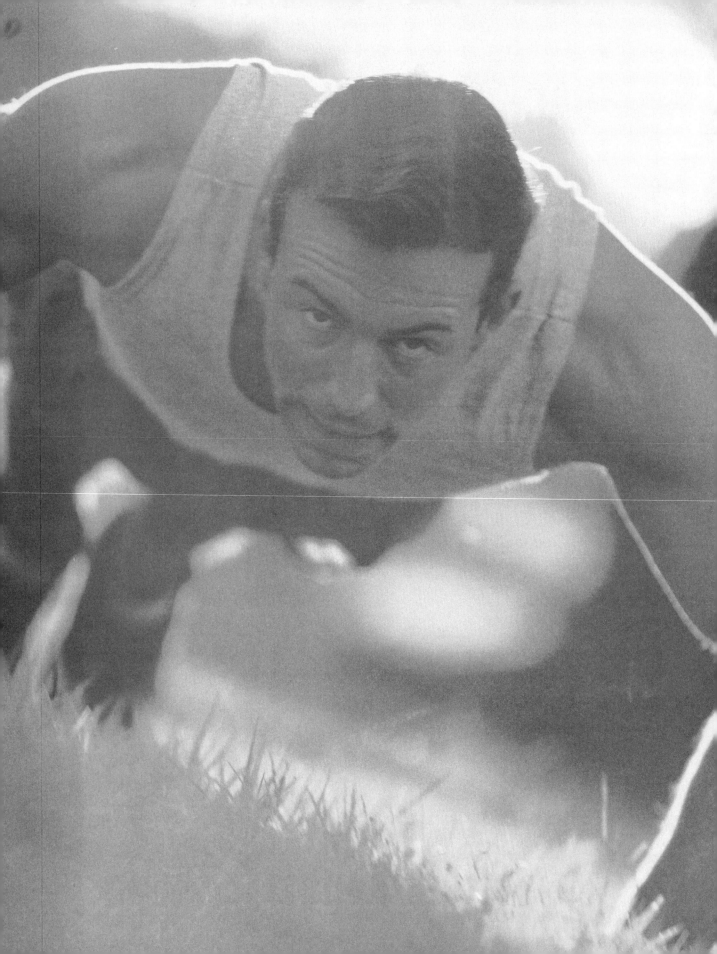

Chapter 4

Chest

Get ready to pump up your chest! In this chapter you'll find all the exercises you need for a chest that is large, chiseled, and strong. For men, it is important to focus on three areas of the chest: the upper chest, with exercises such as the incline dumbbell press; the outer chest, with the incline dumbbell flies; and the inner upper chest, with the incline cable crossovers.

Make sure your form is perfect: always consciously focus and contract the muscles in your chest while maintaining postural alignment and proper form during all of the exercises.

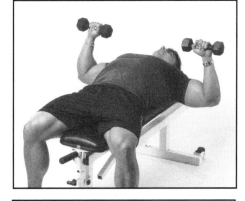

THE BODY SCULPTING BIBLE FOR

CHEST & ARMS

INCLINE DUMBBELL OR BARBELL BENCH PRESS

The incline dumbbell press targets your upper chest muscles. Performing this exercise with dumbbells requires your stabilizer muscles to work to keep the weights balanced. There are two versions of this exercise: one with dumbbells, one with barbells. The dumbbell version requires more control, which helps to strengthen and develop the helper muscles of the chest and shoulders.

TECHNIQUE AND FORM

1 With dumbbells on your thighs, thrust one leg up, leveraging one dumbbell up to your chest.

2 Immediately thrust the second dumbbell upward at the same time as you allow momentum and the dumbbells to guide you back into an inclined position. Use your abdominal muscles to ease you into position.

3 Press the weights straight up to the ceiling. Keep your chest lifted, your elbows out and wide, and your forearms perpendicular to the floor.

4 Lower the weights slowly, making sure your body remains in good alignment.

5 Repeat for the desired number of repetitions.

6 If you are performing the barbell version of this exercise, position yourself on the incline bench and have someone assist you with grasping the barbell. Continue with step 3.

TRAINER'S TIPS

As you perform the exercise, make sure that you pull your shoulder blades back against the bench (this is called retraction). This allows your chest to do more work than your shoulders.

At the top of the movement you have the option of touching the dumbbells together and squeezing your chest or of pressing the weights straight up. As a variation, you can also turn your palms toward each other at the top of the movement.

INCLINE DUMBBELL OR BARBELL BENCH PRESS

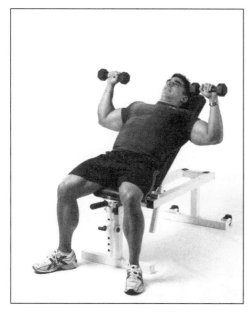
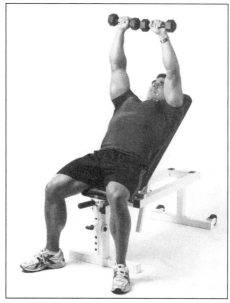
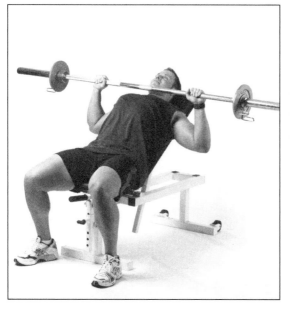
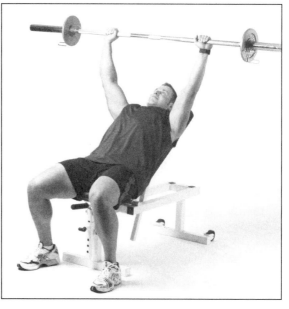

DUMBBELL OR BARBELL BENCH PRESS

This exercise focuses on the muscles in the middle of your chest. There are two versions of this exercise: one with dumbbells, one with barbells. The dumbbell version requires more control, which helps to strengthen and develop the helper muscles of the chest and shoulders.

TECHNIQUE AND FORM

1 With dumbbells on your thighs, thrust one leg up, leveraging one dumbbell up to your chest.

2 Immediately thrust the second dumbbell upward at the same time as you allow momentum and the dumbbells to guide you back into a lying position. Use your abdominal muscles to ease you into position.

3 Keep your back flat by pulling your abdominals in.

4 Beginning from a position where your elbows are slightly lower than the bench, press the weights straight up toward the ceiling, keeping your chest lifted, your elbows out and wide, and your forearms parallel to the floor.

5 Lower the weights slowly, making sure you keep your back pressed into the bench.

6 If you are performing the barbell version of this exercise, position yourself on the incline bench and have someone assist you with grasping the barbell. Continue with step 3.

TRAINER'S TIPS

As you perform the exercise, make sure that you pull your shoulder blades back against the bench (this is called retraction). This allows your chest to do more work than your shoulders.

At the top of the movement you have the option of touching the dumbbells together and squeezing your chest or of pressing them straight up. As a variation, you can also turn your palms toward each other at the top of the movement.

Variety is the spice of exercise, so try the exercise different ways to keep your muscles alert and challenged. Always keep your elbows perpendicular to the floor.

DUMBBELL OR BARBELL BENCH PRESS

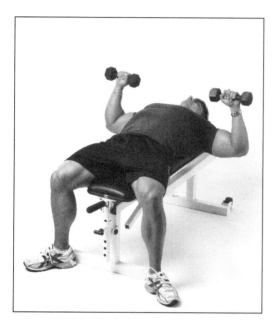
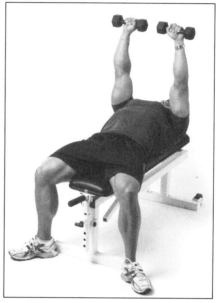
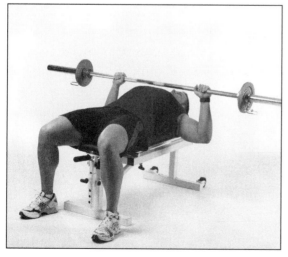
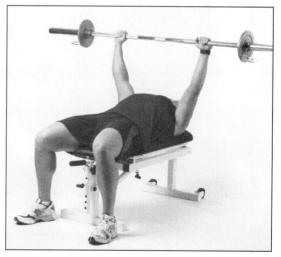

INCLINE DUMBBELL FLY

This exercise focuses on your upper chest muscles, to give you a broad, built look.

TECHNIQUE AND FORM

1 Position yourself on an incline bench, with your shoulder blades retracted (pulled back) and your palms facing forward to increase upper–chest stimulation. Keep your lower back pressed against the bench.

2 Exhale as you squeeze the weights toward each other in an arc–like movement (imagine yourself hugging a tree).

3 At the top of the movement consciously contract your chest muscles as hard as you can.

4 Lower the weights while maintaining proper alignment.

5 Repeat for the desired number of repetitions.

TRAINER'S TIPS

To maintain focus on the chest muscles and minimize involvement of the triceps, as you perform the fly, bend and lock your elbows in place throughout the movement.

To prevent injury to your rotator cuff, as you reach the bottom of the movement do not let the backs of your arms go too far below the bench.

INCLINE DUMBBELL FLY

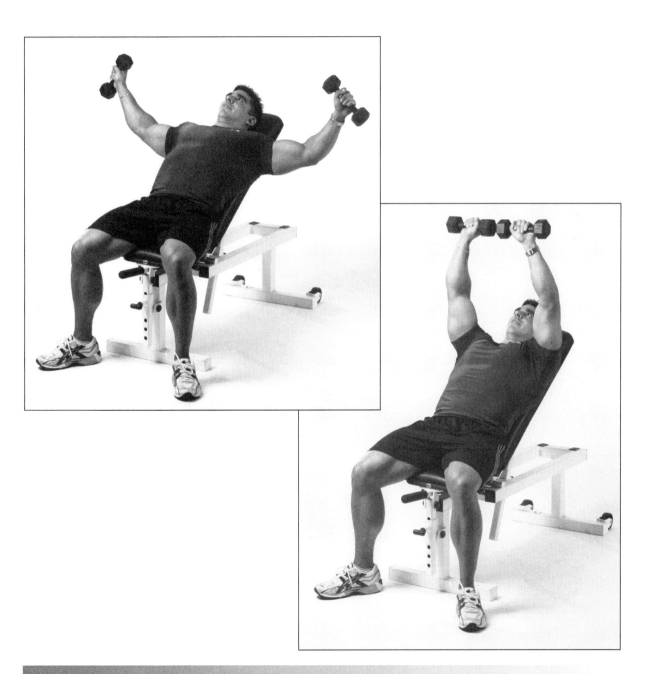

DUMBBELL FLY

This exercise is very similar to the incline version, but it targets more of the midsection of the chest rather than the upper chest.

TECHNIQUE AND FORM

1 Lie flat on a bench, with your back pressed firmly into the bench. Your palms should face each other and your arms should be bent.

2 As you exhale, bring your arms together directly over your chest in an arc–like movement.

3 At the top of the movement consciously contract your chest muscles as hard as you can.

4 Lower the weights while maintaining proper alignment.

5 Repeat for the desired number of repetitions

TRAINER'S TIPS

To maintain focus on the chest muscles and minimize involvement of the triceps, lock your elbow joints in place as you perform the fly.

To prevent injury to your rotator cuff, as you reach the bottom of the movement do not let the backs of your arms go too far below the bench.

Make sure that your lower back stays pressed against the bench; if you find that you are lifting up, it may be an indication that the weight you are lifting is too heavy.

DUMBBELL FLY

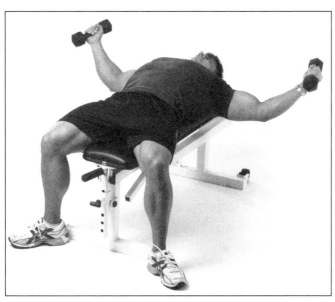

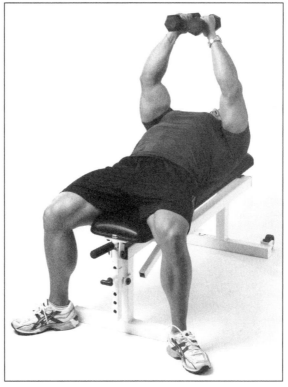

INCLINE CABLE FLY

The cable fly is similar to the dumbbell fly, but you get some added advantage because the cables enable you to maintain resistance throughout the entire range of movement. The incline version helps recruit more fibers in the upper chest.

FREE WEIGHT ALTERNATIVE: Incline Dumbbell Fly

TECHNIQUE AND FORM

1 Set the pin to the desired resistance and attach the handles to the cables. Position an incline bench in the middle of the machine.

2 Sit on the bench and take hold of the handles.

3 Exhale and bring the handles in over your chest in an arc–like motion, with your arms bent.

4 Slowly return to the start position.

5 Repeat for the desired number of repetitions.

TRAINER'S TIPS

✪ Make sure that you contract your chest muscles as hard as possible when the handles are over your chest.

✪ When you release the contraction try not to stretch the arms too far before beginning the next repetition.

INCLINE CABLE FLY

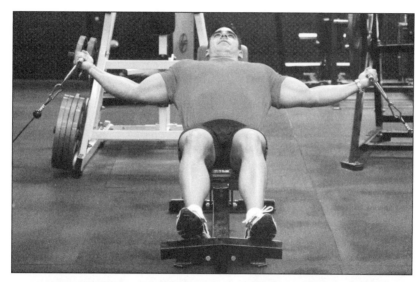

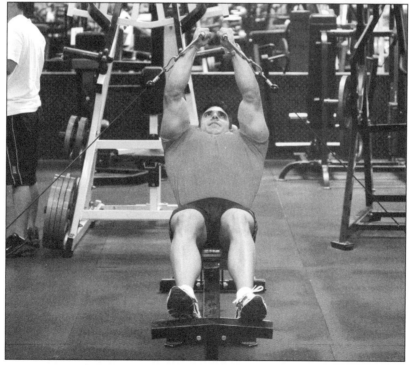

DUMBBELL PULLOVER

The pullover can focus more on your back or chest muscles, depending on the arm technique used and the positioning of your body. This version targets your chest.

TECHNIQUE AND FORM

1 Lie on a flat bench with only your neck and upper back resting against the bench and with your hips positioned well below your rib cage.

2 Lift a dumbbell overhead and hold it at arm's length in front of your face.

3 Slowly lower the weight past your head in an arc–like movement, keeping your arms bent at the elbows to accentuate toning in your chest. Make sure that your hips do not rise when you lower the weight.

4 When you reach a fully stretched position, hold for a second and then begin lifting the weight back up in an arc until you reach your starting position.

TRAINER'S TIPS

If you experience shoulder pain during this exercise, stop immediately.

Make sure that you don't raise your hips as you lower the weight.

DUMBBELL PULLOVER

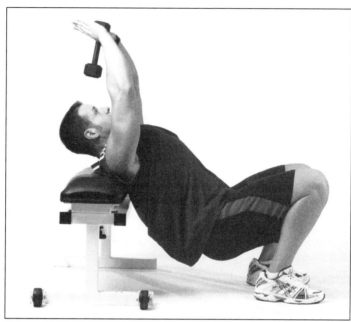

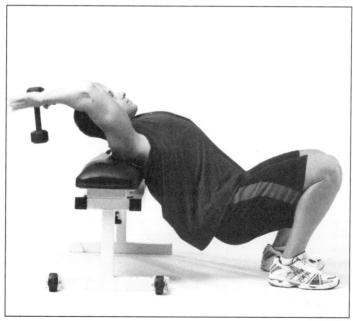

CHEST DIP

The chest dip focuses on the lower chest and serratus muscles. If you find the dips too difficult to do off parallel bars, try using a machine such as the Gravitron, which counter–balances a portion of your body weight.

TECHNIQUE AND FORM

1 Place your hands on parallel bars. Lock out your arms and raise yourself up onto the bars. Bend your legs at the knees and hook your feet over one another.

2 With your body suspended from the floor, lower yourself from the lock out position, while at the same time leaning forward. (The more forward you lean, the more you work your chest).

3 Lower yourself until the backs of your arms are parallel or slightly beyond parallel with the floor.

4 At the bottom position, slowly and smoothly begin to press your body back up, maintaining your alignment.

5 Once at the top position immediately lower back into the bottom position.

6 Repeat for the desired number of repetitions.

TRAINER'S TIPS

✪ There is no rest either at the top or bottom positions; this exercise involves continual movement.

✪ Focus all of your attention on your chest muscles during this exercise to increase involvement of the chest and maintain proper alignment.

✪ This is an advanced chest exercise; you may only be able to do a few reps initially—and remember, if parallel bars are too tough, use a machine that provides assistance with the resistance.

CHEST DIP

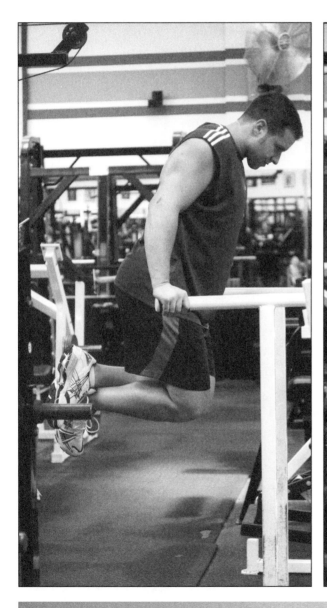 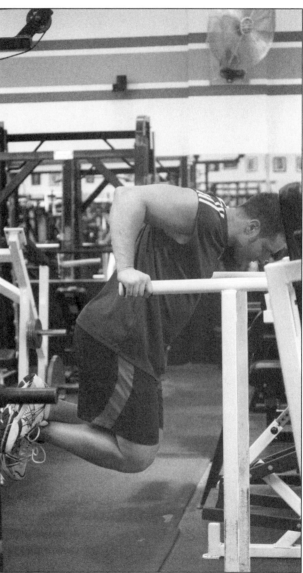

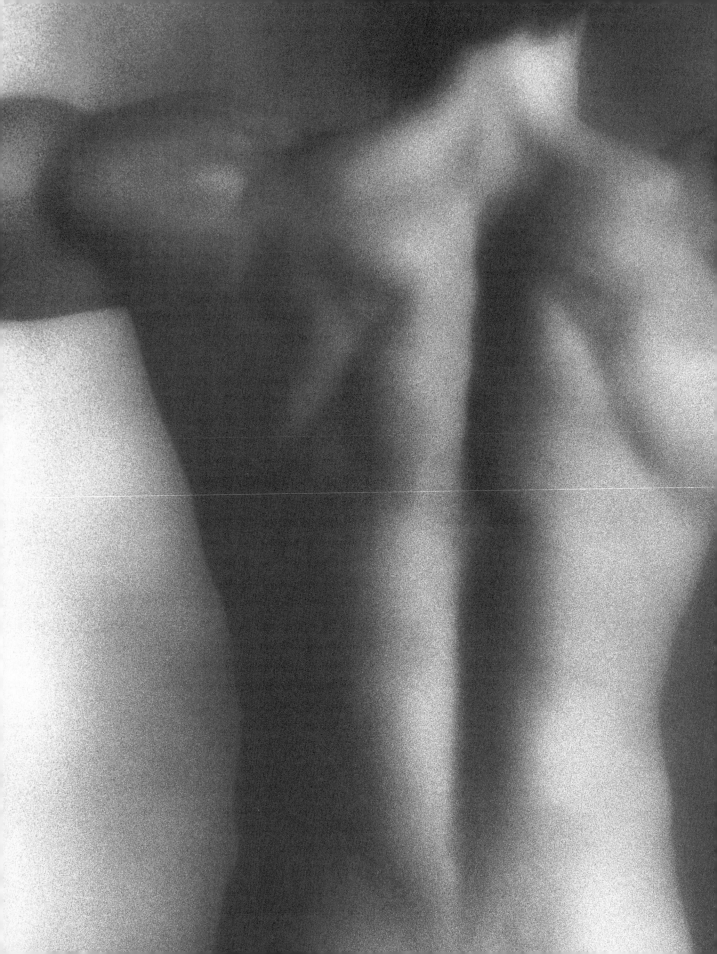

Chapter 5

Back and Shoulders

The back comprises many major muscles, which unfortunately often don't get the workout attention they deserve. Remember, a strong, built back will accentuate your entire upper body as well as making your waist appear smaller! Depending on the grip you choose in an exercise (for example, wide or narrow), you will be concentrating on different areas of a muscle group.

Just as a developed back gives the appearance of a smaller waist, well–defined shoulders provide the illusion of bigger arms. It is important to work all three heads of the shoulder (the anterior, medial, and posterior muscles) in order to achieve a sculpted, three–dimensional appearance.

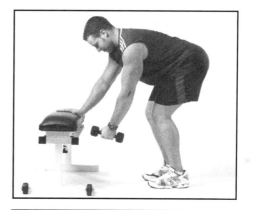

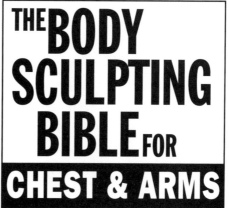

THE **BODY SCULPTING BIBLE** FOR **CHEST & ARMS**

LAT PULLDOWN

This machine targets the latissimus dorsi. Secondary emphasis is placed on the mid–back muscles, trapezius, rhomboids and biceps brachii muscles.

FREE WEIGHT ALTERNATIVE: Pull-Up or One-Arm Row

TECHNIQUE AND FORM

1 Select the desired resistance and adjust the height of the thigh supports that prevent your body from moving up.

2 Grasp the wide bar on the overhead pulley with an overhand grip (palms facing down) about 3 inches away from shoulder width.

3 With both arms extended in front of you holding the bar at the chosen grip width, bring your torso back approximately 30 degrees while creating a curvature in your lower back and sticking your chest out. This is your starting position.

4 Exhale and pull the bar down until it touches your upper chest by drawing your shoulders and upper arms down and back. Concentrate on squeezing your back muscles once you reach the fully contracted position and keeping your elbows close to your body. Your upper torso should remain stationary as you lower the bar.

5 After a second in the contracted position, while breathing in, slowly bring the bar back to the starting position with your arms fully extended and the lats fully stretched.

6 Repeat for the desired number of repetitions.

TRAINER'S TIPS

The only body parts moving should be the arms as they move the pulley toward your chest. Your back and head should always remain stationary, avoiding any type of swinging that could damage your lower back.

Make sure you bring the bar to your chest, not your stomach.

LAT PULLDOWN

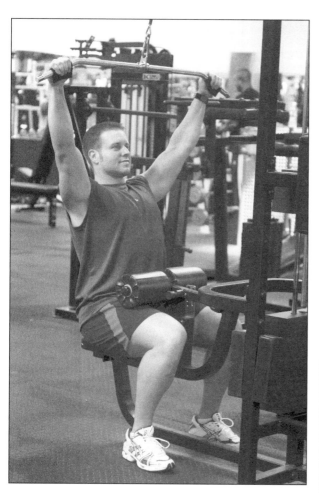

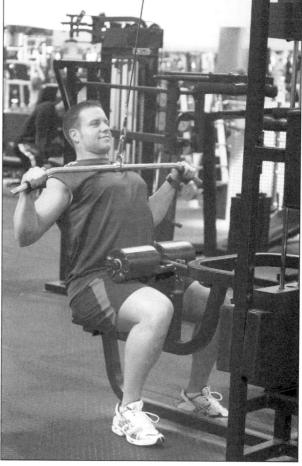

ROW MACHINE

This machine targets the mid–back muscles along with the latissimus dorsi. Secondary emphasis is placed on the trapezius, rhomboids, and biceps brachii muscles.

FREE WEIGHT ALTERNATIVE: One–Arm Row (Palms Facing Torso and Forward)

TECHNIQUE AND FORM

1   Sit on the machine and position your chest against the pad. Depending on the machine used, you may need to adjust the length of the chest pad and the height of the seat to allow your arms to be perpendicular to your torso (at a 90–degree angle) when you grasp the handle bars.

2   Select the desired resistance and grasp the handle bars with a neutral grip (palms facing each other; thumb pointing toward the ceiling). Your arms should be extended in front of you and your shoulders should be stretched. This will be your starting position.

3   Using your back muscles and not your arms, pull the machine lever back towards you until your elbows are past your back and your shoulders are pulled back. Hold the contracted position for a second. Breathe out as you perform this movement.

4   Return to the starting position as you breathe in and repeat for the desired number of repetitions.

TRAINER'S TIPS

✪   To maximize back muscle stimulation, it is important that you adjust the machine so that your arms are at a 90–degree angle from your torso. If your arms are too high, the biceps will take the brunt of the work.

✪   Control the machine at all times and concentrate on using your back muscles rather than your arms.

✪   The movement can also be performed with a palms–down grip or a palms–up grip. This just slightly changes the angle of stimulation.

ROW MACHINE

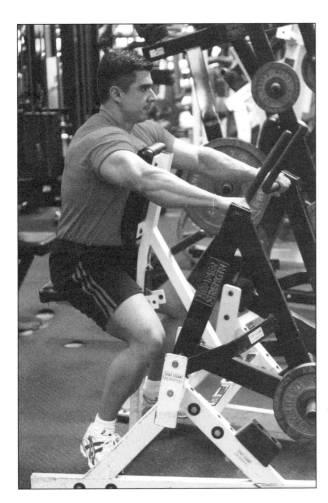

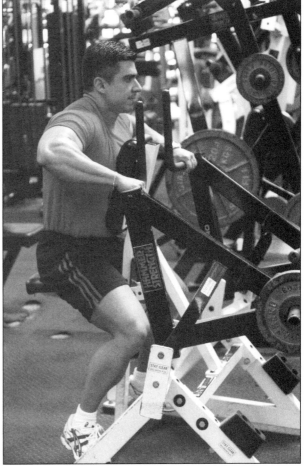

PULLOVER

The pullover can focus more on your back or chest muscles, depending on the arm technique used and the positioning of your body. This version targets your back.

TECHNIQUE AND FORM

1 Lie on a flat bench with only your neck and upper back resting against the bench and with your hips positioned parallel to your rib cage.

2 Lift a dumbbell overhead and hold it at arms' length in front of your face.

3 Slowly lower the weight past your head in an arc–like movement, keeping your arms straight to accentuate stimulation of back muscles. Make sure that your hips do not rise when you lower the weight.

4 When you reach a fully stretched position, hold for a second and then begin lifting the weight back up in an arc until you reach your starting position.

TRAINER'S TIPS

If you experience shoulder pain during this exercise, stop immediately.

Make sure that you don't raise your hips as you lower the weight.

PULLOVER

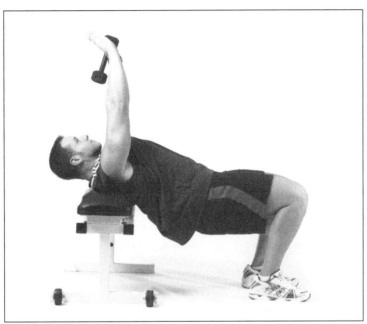

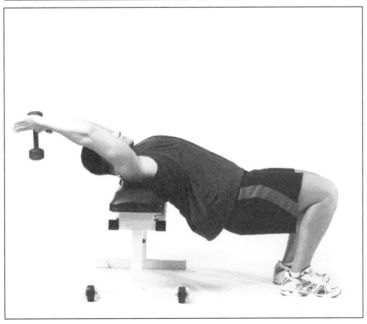

LOW PULLEY CABLE ROW

The Low Pulley Cable Row requires you to stabilize your torso as you perform the row for the lower lats and mid–back muscles.

FREE WEIGHT ALTERNATIVE: One–Arm Row (Palms Facing Torso and Forward)

TECHNIQUE AND FORM

1 Sit on the bench, facing the pulley cables. Lean forward and take hold of the bar.

2 Sit straight up (only a slight lean forward is okay) and bend your knees.

3 With your arms fully extended, retract your shoulders.

4 Keeping your elbows close to your body, pull the bar toward your abdominals, sticking your chest out as far as you can, while striving to sit straight.

5 When the bar reaches your abdominals, squeeze your back muscles hard and hold the position for a count or row.

6 Slowly return to the starting position.

7 Repeat for the desired number of repetitions.

TRAINER'S TIPS

Make sure that you keep your back as straight as possible throughout this exercise, and that your head is in line with your spine.

Make sure that no momentum is involved as you change from the contracted position to the starting position.

LOW PULLEY CABLE ROW

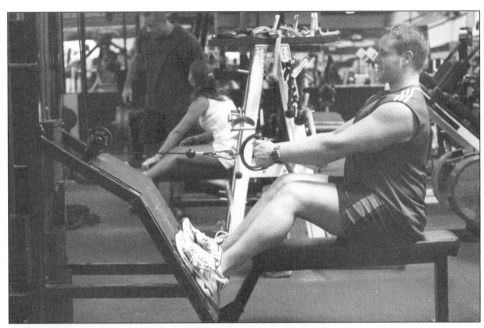

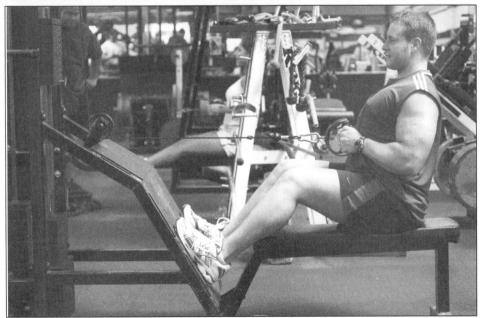

ONE-ARM ROW (PALMS FACING TORSO AND FORWARD)

The One-Arm Row is particularly suited for people with back problems, or who do not yet have strong enough abdominal and other core muscles to lift two weights in good form.

TECHNIQUE AND FORM

1 Place your right hand on a bench or chair for support.

2 Bend at the waist until your upper body is parallel to the bench.

3 Lean into your right hand to help support your body weight. You will be training the left side of your back.

4 Pick up a weight with your left hand so that your palm either faces your torso, or faces forward. Continue to support your back with your right side.

5 Press your left elbow up toward the ceiling. Squeeze and hold in the top position.

6 Slowly lower to starting position.

7 Repeat for desired number of repetitions.

8 Switch sides and perform the same exercise for the right side of you back.

TRAINER'S TIPS

⊗ Be sure to keep your abdominals pulled in tight as you lift the weight.

⊗ Keep your arm right next to your side and your head in line with your spine, and look down or straight ahead throughout the exercise.

⊗ Avoid twisting or turning your torso.

ONE-ARM ROW (PALMS FACING TORSO AND FORWARD)

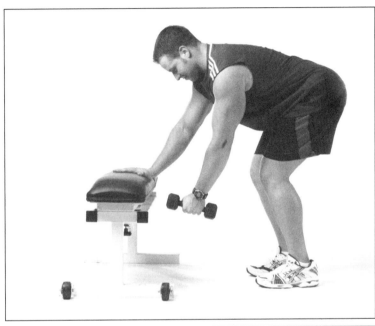

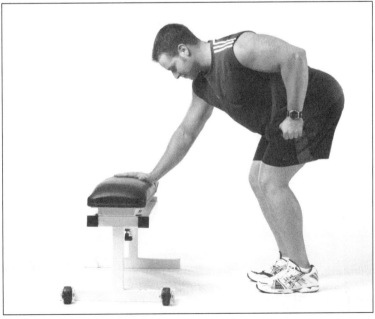

PULL-UP

The pull–up is a tough exercise that requires a great deal of upper body strength. It targets the lats and mid–back muscles. If you find that you cannot pull your own body weight, try a machine such as the Gravitron, which help you to use your body weight. You also can have someone assist you. Or, you can substitute the lat pulldown machine until you've gained enough upper body strength.

TECHNIQUE AND FORM

1 Hold an overhead bar with an overhand grip. Your hands should be about shoulder–width apart. Let your body hang as you contract your abs, bend your legs, and cross your feet.

2 Pull yourself up past the bar, making sure you stick out your chest as much as possible.

3 At the top focus on squeezing and contracting your back muscles hard. Hold for a couple of seconds.

4 As you lower, focus on the back muscles.

5 Repeat for the desired number of repetitions.

TRAINER'S TIPS

Make sure you keep your shoulders depressed (down) while you perform the pull-up.

To attain full range of motion, try to fully straighten your arms at the bottom of the movement.

Target Muscle Groups with Your Grip

Close Grip. Grasp the bar with your hands 4 to 6 inches apart.

Medium Grip. Grasp the bar at shoulder width.

Wide Grip. Grasp the bar 4 to 6 inches beyond shoulder width.

PULL-UP

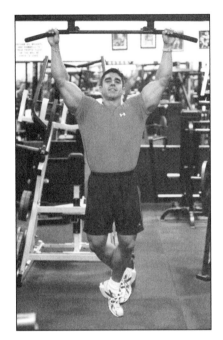

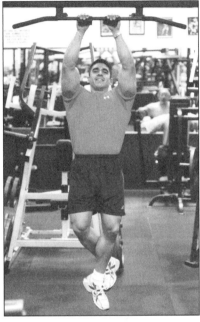

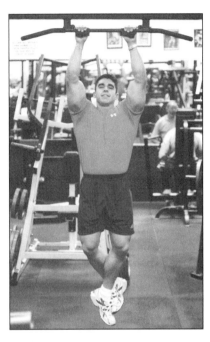

WIDE

NARROW

MEDIUM

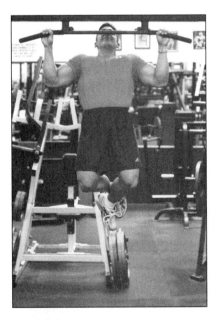

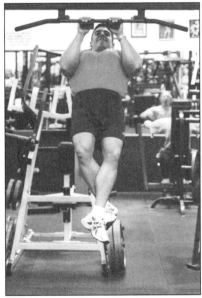

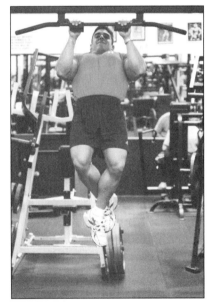

PULL-UP (REVERSE AND NEUTRAL GRIP)

This version of the pull-up targets different musculature in your back: it widens the lower lats and the small serratus muscles on the lower outside of the pecs.

TECHNIQUE AND FORM

1 Take a narrow reverse grip of the bar and hang from it with your arms extended.

2 Bend your lower legs and cross your feet. Stick your chest out and lean your head back.

3 Begin to slowly pull your body up, keeping your elbows close to your body and rowing them behind you.

4 At the top of the movement try to touch your chest to the bar and contract the lat muscles as hard as possible, holding for a couple of seconds.

5 Slowly lower to the start position.

6 Without resting, repeat for the desired number of repetitions.

TRAINER'S TIPS

The key to isolating your back muscles and preventing much stimulation of the biceps is to isometrically contract your lat muscles as you hang (an isometric contraction involves contracting or squeezing (engaging) the muscles without moving).

While you are moving upward, you should feel a strong contraction in your lats.

Lowering slowly with control is essential; it enables you to reap the muscle-building benefits of the negative or eccentric phase of an exercise(the phase during which you elongate your working muscles).

PULL-UP
(REVERSE AND NEUTRAL GRIP)

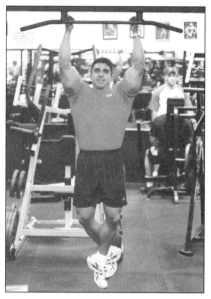
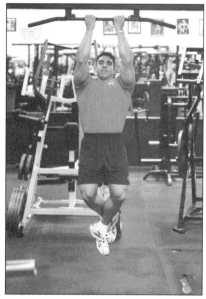

NEUTRAL   **REVERSE**

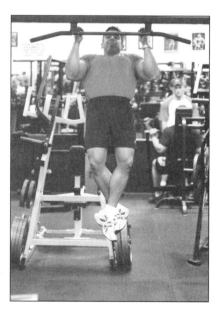
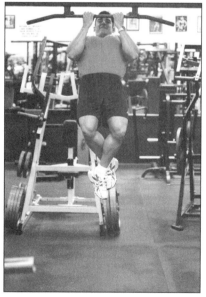

STIFF ARM PULLDOWN

This exercise isolates your back by removing involvement of your biceps. You also are stabilizing and strengthening your core in the standing position.

FREE WEIGHT ALTERNATIVE: Pullover

TECHNIQUE AND FORM

1 Hold onto a pulldown bar with your arms extended and your hands at shoulder width (palms down).

2 With your knees and elbows slightly bent and your wrists locked, press the bar down toward your body in an arc. Move from your shoulder joint, not your elbow.

3 As you lower the bar toward your thighs, concentrate on contracting your lats.

4 When the bar reaches your thighs, hold for a couple of seconds before slowly returning to the start position.

5 Repeat for the desired number of repetitions.

TRAINER'S TIPS

Bending your knees slightly and contracting your abs will help you to stabilize your body during this exercise.

You can also do this exercise using a rope, as shown, keeping your arms stiff as you pull down.

STIFF ARM PULLDOWN

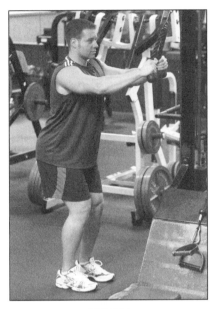

ROPE

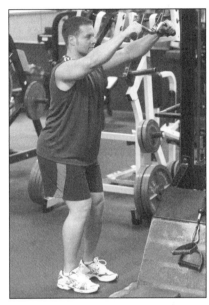

BAR

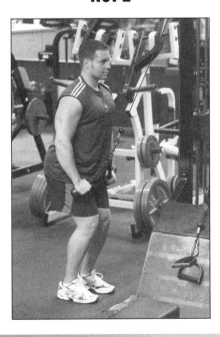

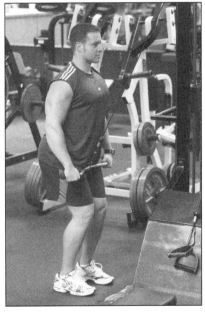

REAR DELT ON MACHINE

This machine targets the rear deltoid most effectively. This is one of the few machines that is almost as effective as its free–weight variety, the Bent-Over Lateral Raise, due to the degree of isolation that it provides.

FREE WEIGHT ALTERNATIVE: Bent–Over Lateral Raises

TECHNIQUE AND FORM

1 Adjust the seat to fit your height and sit on the machine with your torso pressed against the pad. Grasp the handles, which should be at shoulder height.

2 Slightly bend your elbows and rotate your shoulders so that your elbows are to the sides. This is your starting position.

3 Using your rear deltoid muscles, pull the levers apart and to the rear until elbows are just behind your back. There should be a slight bend at the elbows. Exhale as you perform this movement and hold the contraction for a second.

4 Slowly return to the starting position as you inhale.

5 Repeat for the desired number of repetitions.

TRAINER'S TIPS

To maximize rear deltoid involvement, make sure your elbows do not drop below the shoulders. If you let the elbows drop, you begin to use more back muscles to perform the movement.

REAR DELT ON MACHINE

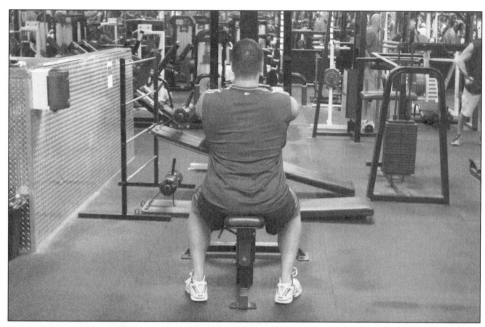

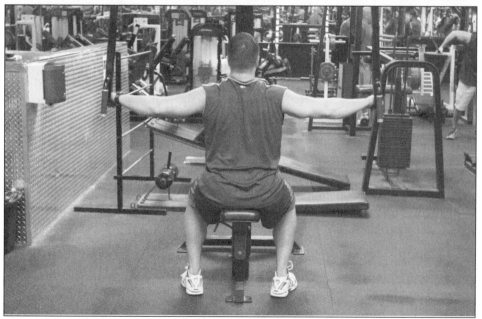

UPRIGHT ROW

This exercise works not only your shoulders, but your upper back (trapezius muscles) as well. You can use weights or a cambered (E–Z curl) bar to begin. The swivel action and curved handles of the E–Z curl bar make it easier on your wrists and shoulders.

TECHNIQUE AND FORM

1 Stand in a neutral alignment (with your body straight, head in line with your spine, knees slightly bent and shoulder–width apart, and a natural curve in your lower back). Hold a weight in each hand with your palms facing the fronts of your thighs.

2 Exhale and lift the dumbbells up toward your chest by bending your elbows. Lift only as high as your chest to avoid hurting your shoulders.

3 Return to starting position and repeat for desired number of repetitions.

TRAINER'S TIPS

Keep your elbows out and higher than the weights as you lift.

Pull your shoulder blades back as you lift the dumbbells.

Concentrate on moving your upper arm and squeezing your shoulder and upper back muscles. This will stimulate the shoulder and upper back muscles more effectively.

Do not use excessive weight for this exercise or you will risk straining your rotator cuff muscles. You will probably need to go lighter than with other exercises for your arms.

UPRIGHT ROW

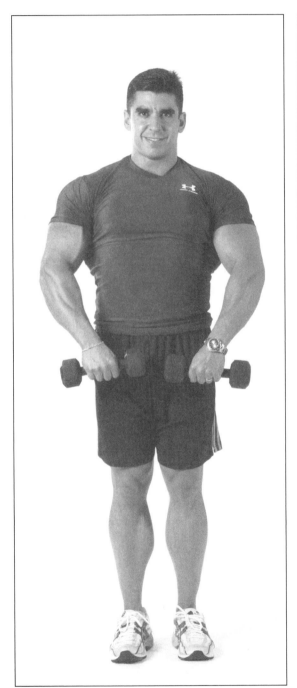
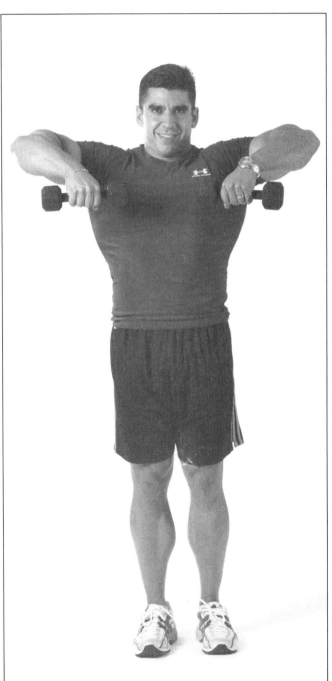

CABLE LATERAL

Using the cables to perform laterals provides resistance during the positive and negative phases of your repetition.

FREE WEIGHT ALTERNATIVE: Dumbbell Side Lateral

TECHNIQUE AND FORM

1 Place the pins at the desired weights in the cable machine.

2 Standing in the center of the cables, slightly lean forward from your hips, still maintaining erect posture. Keep your knees bent and your abdominals engaged. Hold a handle in each hand.

3 Pull the handles in until your arms cross under your chest. This is your starting position.

4 Extend your arms in an upward arc–like movement, until they are parallel to the floor.

5 At the top position, hold for a couple of seconds before returning to the crossed position.

6 Repeat for the desired number of repetitions.

TRAINER'S TIPS

✪ You may need to use lighter weights than usual for this exercise; if you feel any pain in your neck; that is an indication that the weight you are lifting may be too heavy.

✪ Keep your head in line with your spine throughout this exercise.

CABLE LATERAL

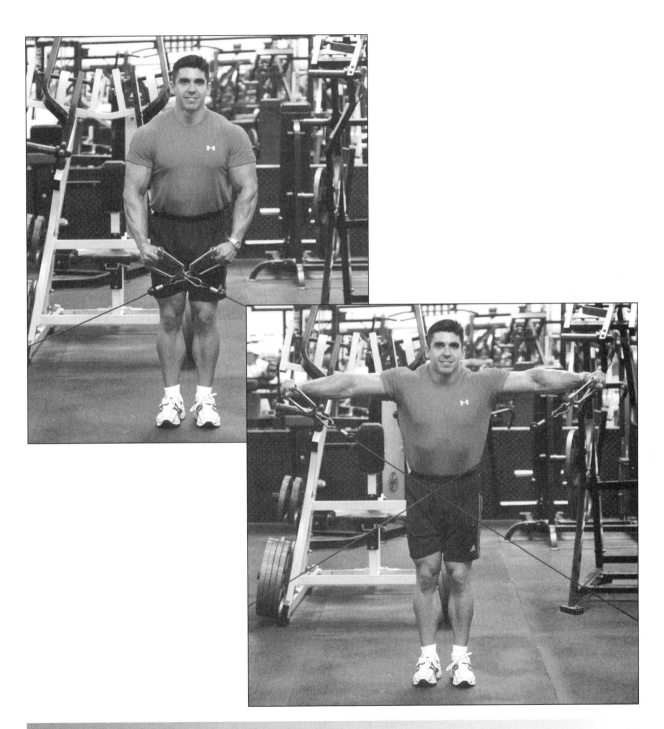

DUMBBELL SIDE LATERAL

The dumbbell lateral raise to the side isolates the side deltoid. Because this is a relatively small muscle, you will need to use lighter weight to ensure perfect form.

TECHNIQUE AND FORM

1 Stand in neutral position with a dumbbell in each hand. Keeping your knees slightly bent, exhale, and lift your arms out to the side—keeping them as straight as possible—until they are slightly higher than parallel to the floor.

2 At the top of the movement, hold for a second or two before slowly lowering the dumbbells to your starting position.

3 Repeat for the desired number of repetitions.

TRAINER'S TIPS

If you bend your arms at the elbows when you raise the weights you will not get maximum deltoid stimulation. If you find you cannot lift the weights without bending your arms, you need to use lighter weights.

If you find that your back is swaying, you need to use lighter weights.

DUMBBELL SIDE LATERAL

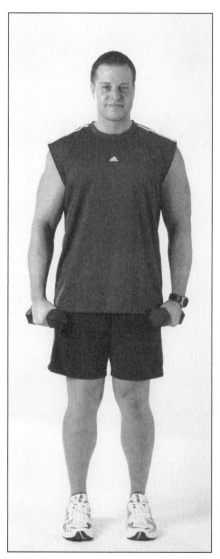
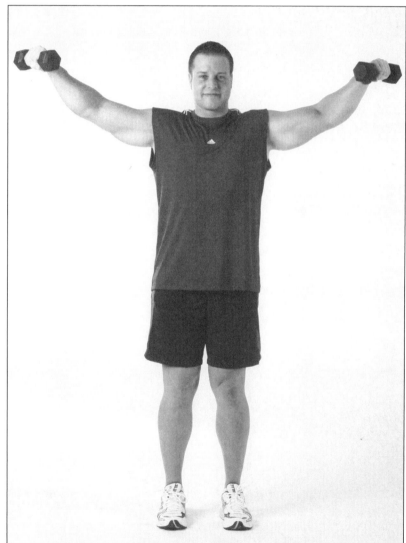

MILITARY PRESS

The military press works the front and side of the shoulders. It's a great exercise that not only challenges the shoulders, but works on your balance and stability too.

TECHNIQUE AND FORM

1 Stand in neutral position, with your knees slightly bent and your feet shoulder–width apart for support. Hold a dumbbell in each hand over your shoulders. Your palms should face forward and your elbows should be at a 90–degree angle.

2 Exhale as you press the dumbbells straight up in a controlled, smooth motion.

3 Once you reach the top (your arms should remain slightly bent at the elbows), hold for a moment before lowering slowly down back to the 90–degree angle.

TRAINER'S TIPS

❖ Throughout the exercise make sure you keep your arms wide, your head in line with your spine, and your back straight.

❖ If you find you are swaying either forward or backward, you need to adjust your form, or go lighter on the weights.

❖ Concentrate on keeping your elbows as wide as possible throughout the exercise.

❖ It is unnecessary to touch the weights together at the top of the movement—this may actually injure your rotator cuff muscles.

MILITARY PRESS

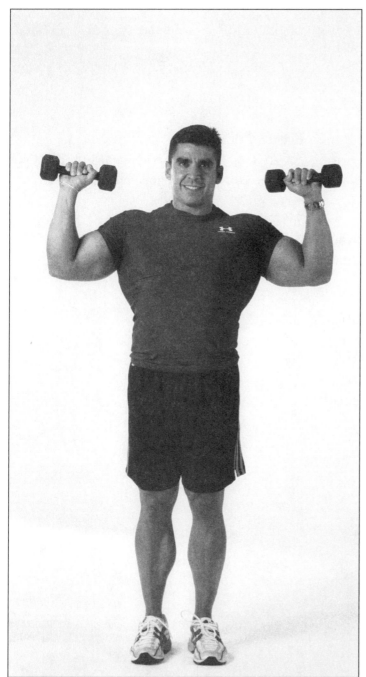
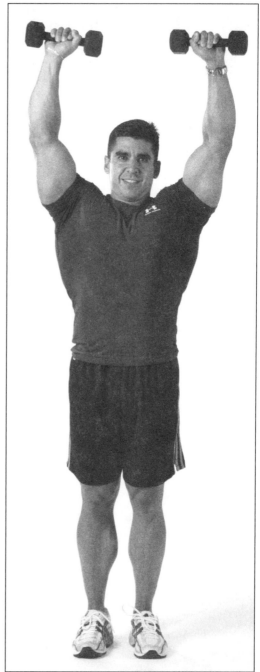

BENT-OVER LATERAL RAISE

This exercise develops the back muscles of your shoulder (the rear deltoids) and helps to give your shoulders a three–dimensional appearance.

TECHNIQUE AND FORM

1 Stand in neutral position, then bend over at your hips. Bend your knees, and keep your back straight and parallel to the floor.

2 Lift the dumbbells out to the sides of your body—to shoulder height—keeping your arms slightly bent at the elbows.

3 When you reach the top position, hold it momentarily before returning to the start position.

4 Repeat for desired number of repetitions.

TRAINER'S TIPS

To help keep your back straight throughout the exercise, pull your abdominals in tight.

BENT-OVER LATERAL RAISE

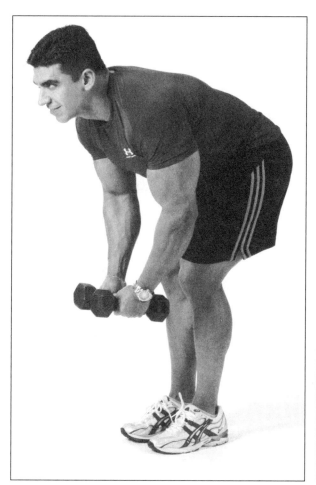
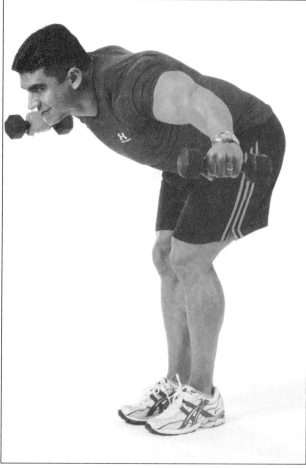

ROTATOR CUFF

The four small muscles of the rotator cuff need strengthening, or they are prone to injury.

TECHNIQUE AND FORM

1 Stand in neutral position, holding a light weight in each hand.

2 Bend your arms so that the upper and lower arms are at a 90-degree angle, with your arms parallel to the floor, extended before you.

3 Exhale and rotate at your shoulders so that your hands rise above your elbows and your palms face front.

4 Slowly return to the start position.

5 Repeat for the desired number of repetitions.

TRAINER'S TIPS

✪ Make sure you maintain the 90–degree angle in the arms throughout the range of motion.

✪ You will need to use weight that is markedly lighter for this exercise than for other arm exercises.

ROTATOR CUFF

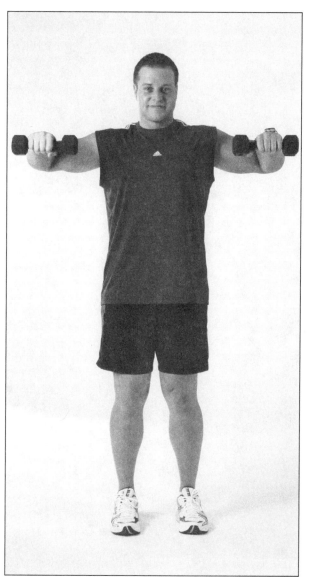

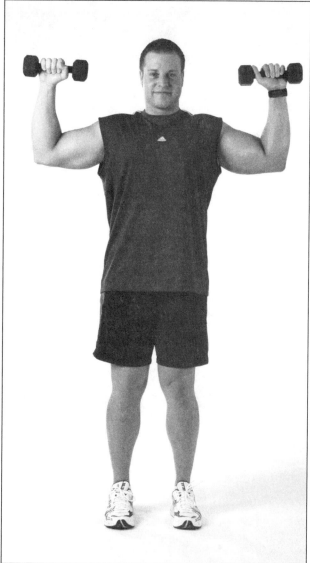

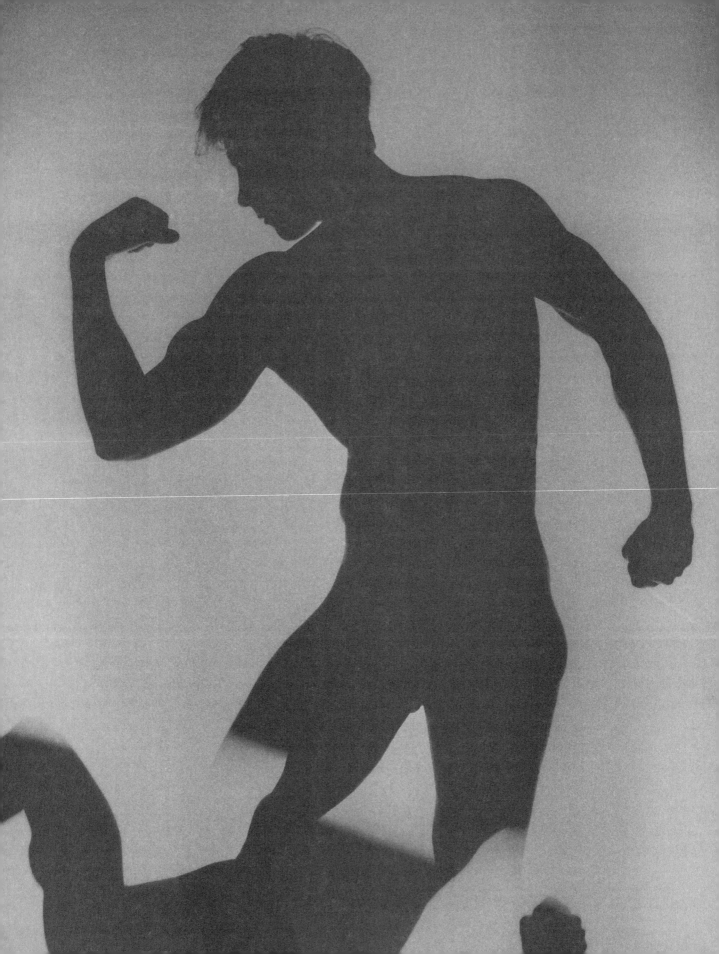

Chapter 6
Biceps and Triceps

Bulging biceps and tight triceps are yours for the taking. The exercises that follow home in on the major muscles in the front and back of your arms. While you work these muscles as secondary movers when you perform chest and back exercises, the ones included here are designed to enlist the biceps and triceps as primary movers. Bear in mind that your triceps muscles comprise two-thirds of your arms, so you need to focus on them as well (and not just on the biceps) if you want well-balanced, sculpted arms.

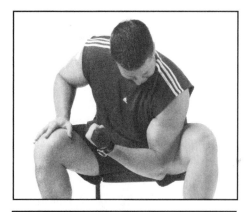

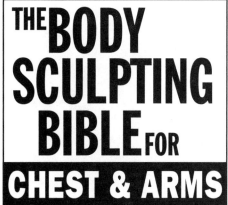

THE BODY SCULPTING BIBLE FOR CHEST & ARMS

6

DUMBBELL CURL OR ALTERNATE DUMBBELL CURL

Dumbbell curls isolate the biceps most effectively and also protect your wrist from undue stress like that created by a barbell curl. In the alternate curl version you perform one rep with your right arm, then one with your left arm, and continue alternating in this way for the desired number of repetitions.

TECHNIQUE AND FORM

1 Stand in neutral alignment with your abs held in and a natural curve to your spine. Hold a dumbbell in each hand. Your arms are slightly bent at the elbows and your palms face out.

2 Slowly curl the dumbbells up toward your shoulders, without moving your elbows.

3 Once you reach the top position, hold for a moment, contracting your biceps are hard as you can, before returning to the starting position.

4 Repeat immediately and perform the desired number of repetitions.

TRAINER'S TIPS

Be careful not to sway back or forward while executing the curl; if you do, you may be using weight that is too heavy.

Make sure your arms are not locked out when in the down position; this will place too much pressure on your biceps and make you vulnerable to injury.

Perform the bicep curls with a great deal of control, being careful not to use momentum to lift the weights.

DUMBBELL CURL OR ALTERNATE DUMBBELL CURL

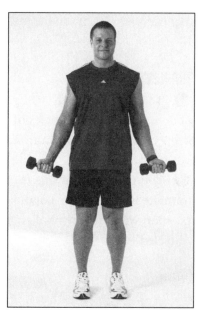
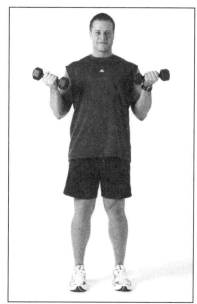

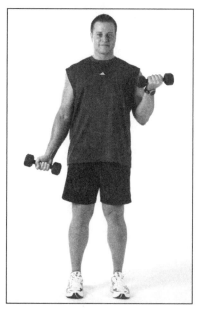
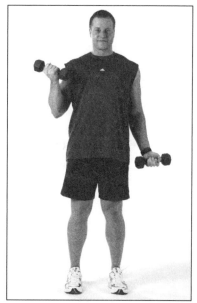

HAMMER CURL WITH ROTATION

The Hammer Curl with Rotation works the outer biceps, thus making your arms look wider, and also target your forearms. It is similar to the Dumbbell Curl, only this exercise is performed with your palms facing each other. In this exercise, you also add a rotation of the arm (supination) to recruit more muscle fibers. You can also perform this exercise alternating arms as you curl.

TECHNIQUE AND FORM

1 Stand in a neutral alignment (with your body straight, head in line with your spine, knees slightly bent and shoulder–width apart, and a natural curve to your lower back). Hold a weight in each hand with your palms facing each other.

2 Exhale and curl the dumbbells up toward your shoulders. As you lift the weights, rotate your arms so that your palms face your shoulders. Make sure you keep your elbows at your sides and pointed at the ground throughout the exercise.

3 At the top position, contract your biceps and forearm muscles as hard as you can and hold for a couple of seconds.

4 Slowly and smoothly return to starting position and repeat for the desired number of repetitions.

TRAINER'S TIPS

To keep your body straight, pull in your abdominal muscles, stick out your chest and keep your shoulders squared.

You can perform this exercise while seated to make it more of an isolation exercise—this position will be more challenging for the biceps muscles.

HAMMER CURL WITH ROTATION

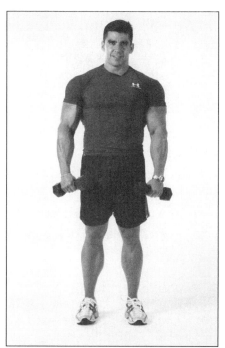
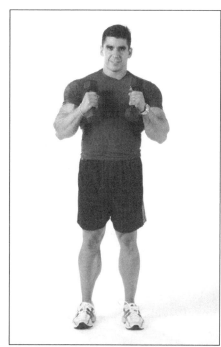
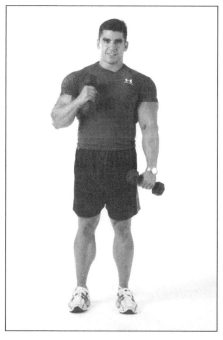
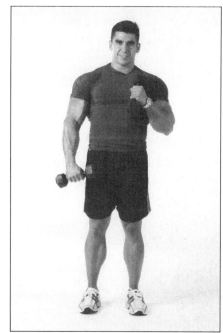

INCLINE HAMMER CURL

The incline hammer curl requires strict form and isolation. This exercise mainly targets the outer biceps and forearms.

TECHNIQUE AND FORM

1 Sit on an incline bench, set to a 45–degree angle.

2 Select two dumbbells of weight that allows you to use proper form.

3 Lean back into the bench so that your back is against the pad. Remain there for the entire exercise.

4 With your palms facing in toward the bench, exhale and curl your arms.

5 Slowly and smoothly lower your weights to the starting position.

6 Repeat for the desired number of repetitions.

TRAINER'S TIPS

✷ Make sure that your elbows remain pointed directly to the floor during this exercise. Do not allow your shoulders to flex forward; this will decrease the stimulation of the biceps.

INCLINE HAMMER CURL

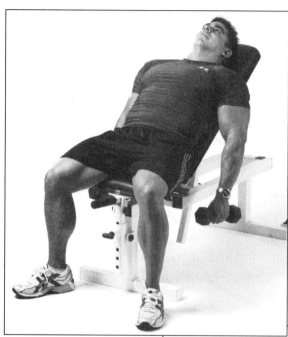

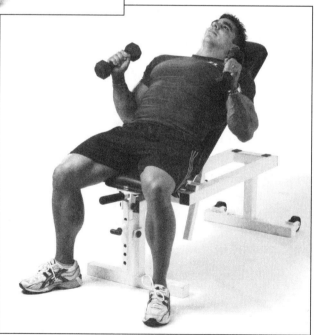

HIGH CABLE CURL

This movement targets the biceps brachii with secondary emphasis on the brachialis.

TECHNIQUE AND FORM

1 Stand in front of a pulldown machine with a bar attached to the pulley.

2 Grab the bar, using a shoulder–wide grip, and position your upper arms so that they are parallel to the floor with the palms facing up. This will be your starting position.

3 Curl the bar toward you until it is close to your forehead. Make sure that as you do so you flex your biceps and exhale. The upper arms should remain stationary and only the forearms should move. Hold for a second on the contracted position.

4 Slowly bring your arms back to the starting position as you inhale.

5 Repeat for the desired amount of repetitions.

TRAINER'S TIPS

When you grab the bar before starting the exercise you may slant your torso a bit backward to maintain good balance.

Your upper arms must remain stationary, as moving them will take off stimulation from the biceps.

HIGH CABLE CURL

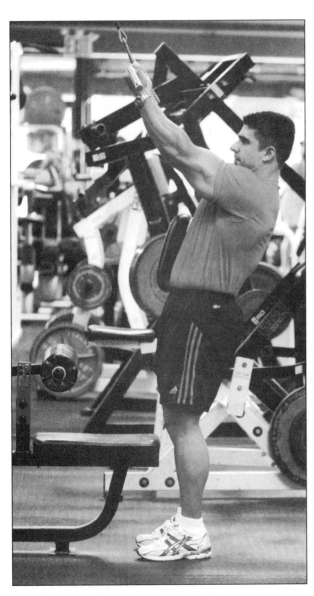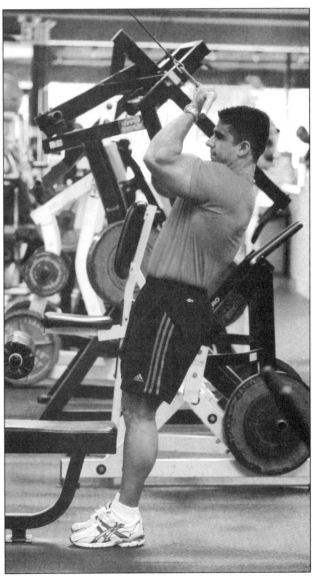

CURL (ARMS TURNED OUT)

Here's a variation of the traditional biceps curl that recruits the biceps muscle fibers from a different angle.

TECHNIQUE AND FORM

1 Begin in a standing position with your abs pulled in, your knees slightly bent and your legs shoulder–width apart for balance and support. Holding a weight in each hand, turn your arms out to your sides.

2 Slowly lift the weights toward your shoulders. In the top position, hold for a couple of seconds.

3 Slowly return to the starting position.

4 Repeat for the desired number of repetitions.

TRAINER'S TIPS

Make sure you keep your elbows in by the sides of your waist throughout the exercise.

When you lower the weights, try not to come into too much of a stretch—this could strain your biceps.

CURL (ARMS TURNED OUT)

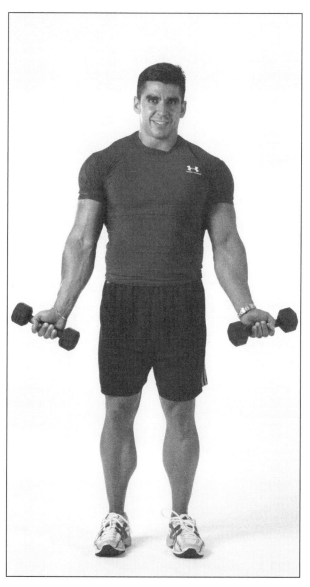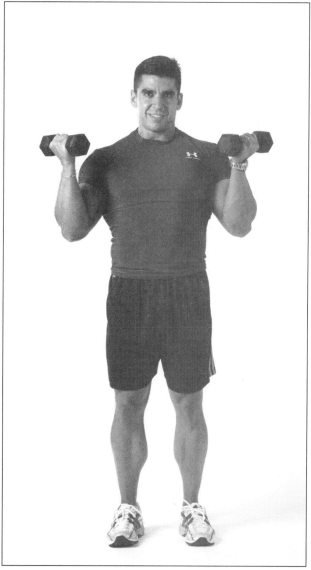

CONCENTRATION CURL

The concentration curl involves intense focus on the contraction of the biceps—something you should do in all of the exercises.

TECHNIQUE AND FORM

1 Maintain a seated position, bend at the hips and hold a weight in one hand.

2 Support your arm by resting your elbow on your thigh.

3 Curl the weight toward your shoulder while you also rotate your wrist. (The arm that you are exercising is extended to begin, while the other arm rests on your thigh.)

4 At the top position, hold for two seconds before slowly lowering back to the starting position.

5 Repeat for the desired number of repetitions. (Switch to other arm)

TRAINER'S TIPS

There is no rest between repetitions; immediately move fluidly from one rep to the next.

CONCENTRATION CURL

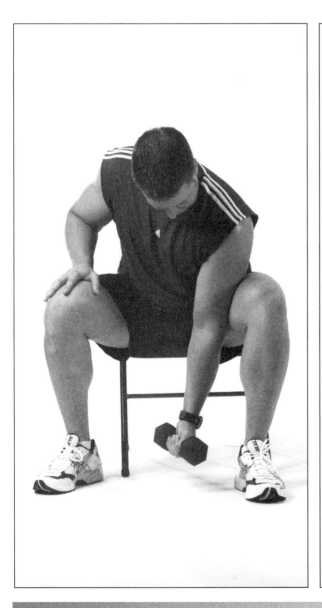
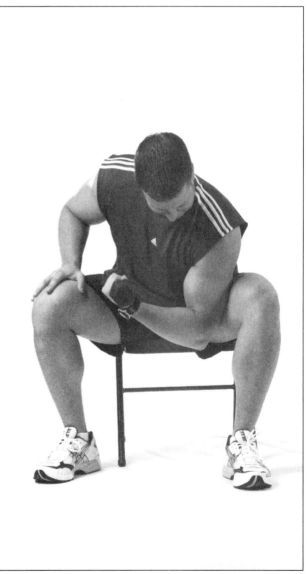

REVERSE E–Z CURL

The reverse E–Z curl targets the brachialis (also known as the outer biceps) and forearm muscles.

TECHNIQUE AND FORM

1 Grasp an E–Z bar with your arms fully straightened and your palms facing in toward your thighs (this is a reverse grip).

2 With your feet shoulder–width apart and your knees slightly bent, exhale and curl the bar up to your shoulders in an arc–like movement concentrating all the while on your forearms and biceps.

3 At the top of the movement, squeeze your biceps as hard as you can; hold for a second or two and then lower to the start position.

4 Repeat for the desired number of repetitions.

TRAINER'S TIPS

◆ Make sure you engage your abdominals and keep your knees bent to avoid recruiting your lower back in this exercise.

◆ Keep your head level—looking straight ahead—for the duration of the exercise.

REVERSE E–Z CURL

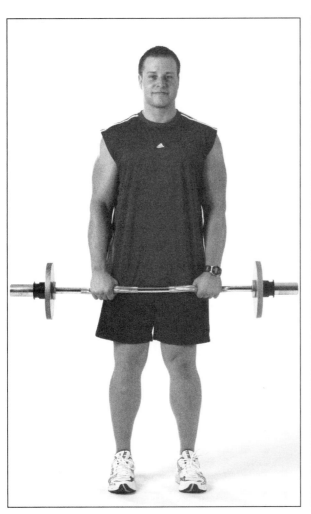

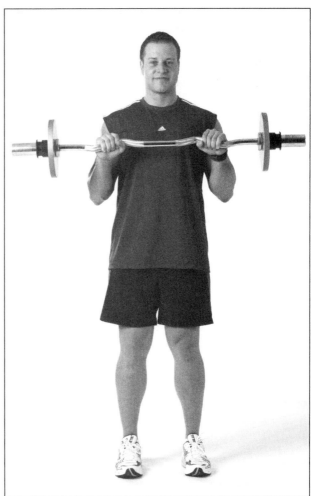

PREACHER CURL

The Preacher Curl develops the lower part of your biceps, helping to build balance in the muscle.

TECHNIQUE AND FORM

1 To perform this movement you will either need a preacher bench or the top of an incline bench.

2 Grab a dumbbell with your right arm and place your upper arm on top of the preacher bench or the incline bench. The dumbbell should be held at shoulder height. This will be your starting position.

3 As you breathe in, slowly lower the dumbbell until your upper arm is extended and the biceps muscle is fully stretched.

4 As you exhale, use the biceps to curl the weight up until your biceps is fully contracted and the dumbbell is at shoulder height. To ensure a full contraction you need to bring your small finger higher than your thumb.

5 Repeat for the desired number of repetitions.

TRAINER'S TIPS

Here are two variations of this exercise: perform it using a low pulley instead of a dumbbell. In this case you will need to position the bench in front of the pulley. You also can use an E–Z bar, but in this case, you cannot just use an incline bench; you will need a preacher bench.

PREACHER CURL

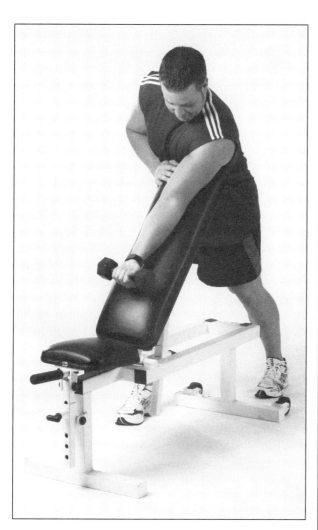

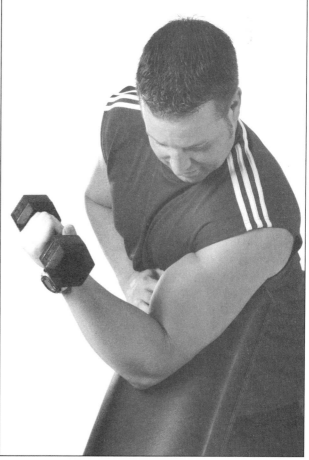

OVERHEAD DUMBBELL TRICEPS EXTENSION

This exercise targets the middle and inner triceps muscles. It can be performed either seated or standing.

TECHNIQUE AND FORM

1 Begin in a seated or standing position. If seated, make sure that your back is flat against the back pad at all times. If standing, make sure that your abs are pulled in and your knees are slightly bent and your legs are shoulder width apart for balance and support.

2 Hold the dumbbell with both hands over your head, grasping it so that you get an even grip with both hands. (This is important; if your grip is uneven, you will be working out one arm more than the other).

3 Lower the dumbbell while keeping your elbows pointed to the ceiling.

4 Exhale as you press the dumbbell back up to the top position.

5 At the top position, contract the triceps as hard as you can and hold for a couple of seconds before lowering.

6 Repeat for desired number of repetitions.

TRAINER'S TIPS

✪ Throughout the exercise, make sure your elbows are in close to your head and pointed up at the ceiling. This ensures full range of motion for the triceps.

✪ When you extend your arms, maintain a slight bend to the elbows to avoid locking out at the joint.

✪ Keep your head in line with your spine throughout the exercise—avoid looking down.

OVERHEAD DUMBBELL TRICEPS EXTENSION

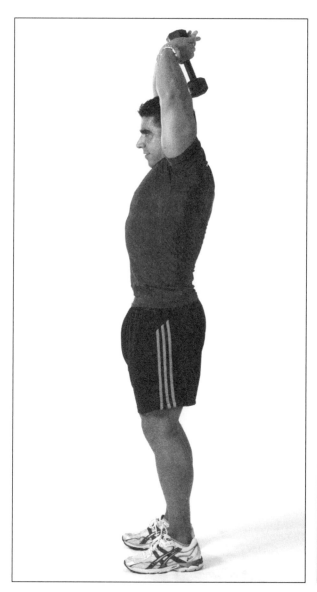
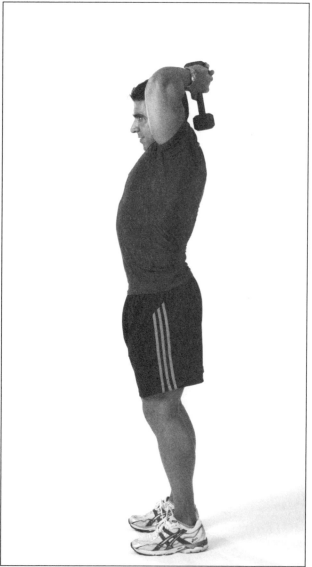

KICKBACK

The classic Kickback sculpts and defines the triceps muscles. Perform this exercise with your arms almost parallel to the floor for maximum muscle recruitment.

TECHNIQUE AND FORM

1 Bend forward so that your back is as close to parallel with the floor as possible. Hold a weight in your right hand. You can support yourself by placing your left hand on a bench.

2 Lift your elbow so that it is higher than your back. Your arm should be bent, with the weight near your shoulder.

3 Exhale and extend your right arm by pressing your forearm behind you.

4 When you reach a near–fully extended position, squeeze the triceps muscles hard and hold for a second or two.

5 Slowly bend your arm so that the weight returns to your shoulder.

6 Repeat for the desired number of repetitions. Switch sides.

TRAINER'S TIPS

Try not to lock out your elbow joint at any point during the exercise. In the extended position, you should come just short of a lockout.

Maintain depression of your shoulder (don't let your shoulder rise to your ear)

Make sure that your upper arm (from the shoulder to the elbow) remains stationary throughout the exercise.

KICKBACK

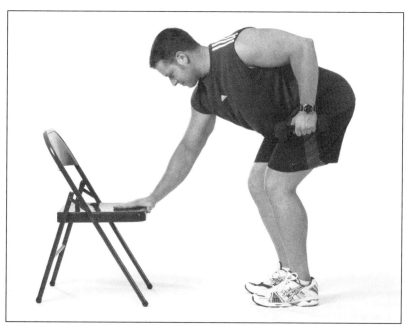

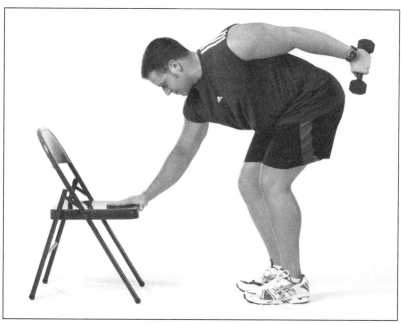

TRICEPS PUSHDOWN

This movement targets the triceps brachii. You may also use a v–bar, short cambered bar attachment, or straight bar for this exercise.

TECHNIQUE AND FORM

1 Attach a rope to a high pulley and grab with an overhand grip (palms facing down) at shoulder width. Standing upright with your torso straight and a very small inclination forward, bring your upper arms close to your body and perpendicular to the floor. Your forearms should be pointing up toward the pulley as you hold the rope. This is your starting position.

2 Using the triceps, bring the rope down until it touches the front of your thighs and your arms are fully extended perpendicular to the floor. Your upper arms should always remain stationary next to your torso and only the forearms should move. Exhale as you perform this movement.

3 Hold after a second at the contracted position, bring the rope slowly up to the starting point. Breathe in as you perform this step.

4 Repeat for the desired number of repetitions.

TRAINER'S TIPS

When you grab the bar or rope before starting the exercise you may slant your torso a bit forward to maintain good balance

It is of utmost importance that your upper arms remain stationary next to your torso as moving them removes stimulation from the triceps.

TRICEPS PUSHDOWN

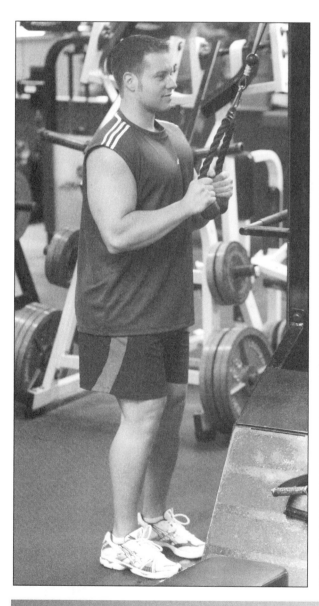
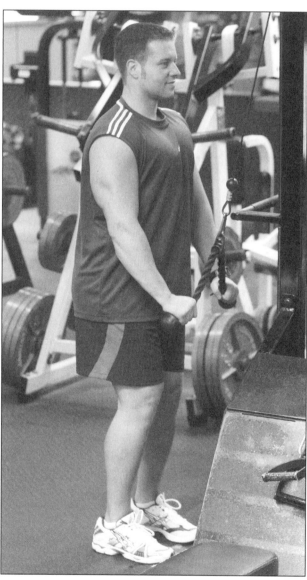

CLOSE GRIP BENCH PRESS

This exercise works both the inner chest and triceps.

TECHNIQUE AND FORM

1 Lie on a bench, with your feet flat on the floor.

2 Lift the bar into place by pressing it up using your chest muscles. Hold it above your head, placing your hands in the outer curved portion of the bar.

3 Slowly lower the bar as if you were doing a bench press, but keep your arms close to your body so that your arms are in direct line with the front of your shoulders.

4 As you lower, keep your arms close to the sides of your body to stimulate the triceps.

5 When you reach the down position, use your triceps to push the bar back to the start position.

6 Squeeze in the top position for one to two seconds.

7 Repeat for the desired number of repetitions.

TRAINER'S TIPS

Keep the movement fluid and smooth throughout the exercise. There is no resting when switching between the lowered and raised positions.

CLOSE GRIP BENCH PRESS

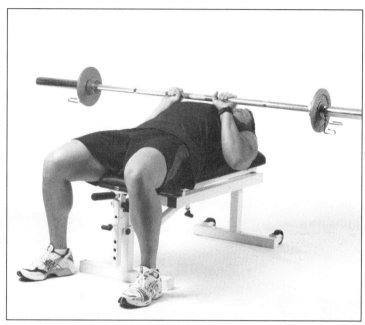

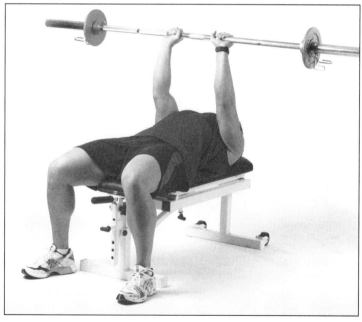

TRICEPS DIP

The triceps dip targets the lower triceps. For this exercise you must use a dip station or machine. Or you may do this exercise off a bench.

TECHNIQUE AND FORM

1 Position yourself on the parallel bars, aligning your body from your head to your toes.

2 Begin in a locked out position, with your arms fully extended and lower yourself, leaning back to keep your body in an upright position.

3 Keep your elbows close to your body to focus on the triceps. You should reach the point where your feet come close to the floor.

4 Immediately push yourself back up.

5 Repeat for the desired number of repetitions.

TRAINER'S TIPS

✪ Keep your abdominal muscles engaged to maintain good form.

✪ Do not lock your elbows in the top position; instead focus on squeezing the triceps muscles as hard as you can for a couple of seconds. Remember your triceps, NOT YOUR ELBOWS, should feel challenged here.

TRICEPS DIP

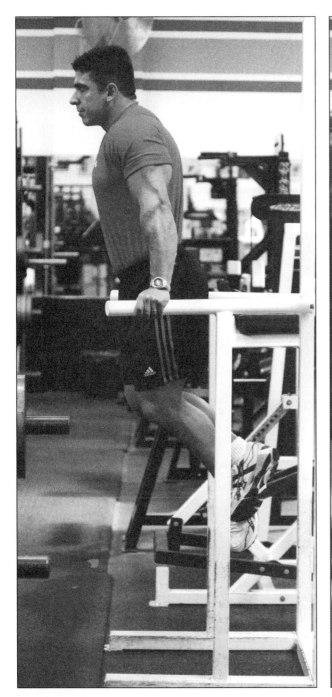
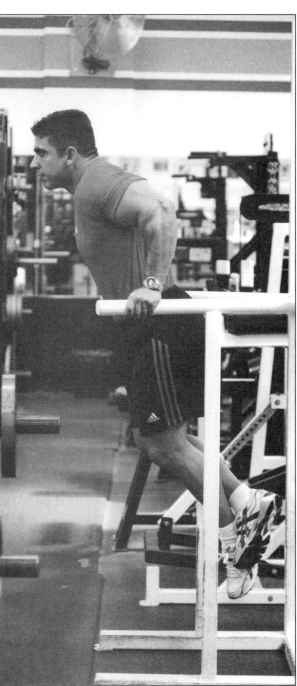

LYING TRICEPS EXTENSION

The triceps are three muscles located at the back of your upper arm; this exercise focuses on the outer muscles.

TECHNIQUE AND FORM

1 Lie on your back and, with a dumbbell in each hand, press your arms toward the ceiling. Your palms should face each other.

2 Bend your elbows to lower the dumbbells toward your head. The upper part of your arms should remain frozen in place—only your forearms move during this exercise.

3 Once the weights come close to your forehead, slowly press them back up to the starting position (with arms extended).

4 Hold that position and squeeze your triceps hard.

5 Repeat for the desired number of repetitions.

TRAINER'S TIPS

At the top of the exercise, contract your triceps as hard as you can and concentrate on them. This will increase stimulation of the triceps.

Even though you are straightening your arms over your head, always maintain a slight bend to your elbows for safety.

LYING TRICEPS EXTENSION

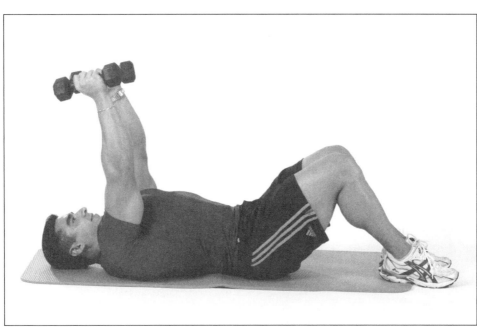

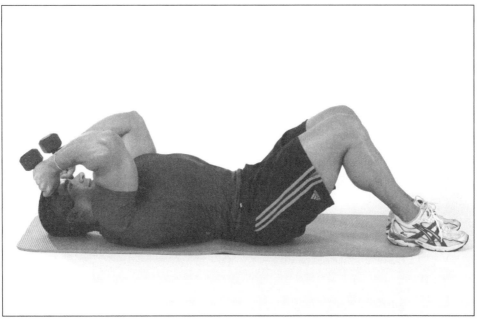

LYING E–Z TRICEPS EXTENSION

This triceps exercise fully stimulates all three muscles of the triceps.

TECHNIQUE AND FORM

1 Set up a cambered bar (E–Z curl bar) with light weight on each side, or use one that is already pre–weighted.

2 Lie on a bench, with your feet flat on the floor. Hold onto the bar, positioning your hands about 8 to 10 inches apart, and bring the bar overhead. Your elbows should point slightly behind you, toward the ceiling at an angle.

3 Slowly lower the bar toward your forehead, keeping your elbows pointed slightly behind you at an angle toward the ceiling.

4 Exhale and straighten the bar, raising it up above your head as you straighten your arms. At the top of the exercise focus on contracting your triceps as hard as you can. Hold for a second before once again bending your arms back down to the starting position.

5 Repeat for the desired number of repetitions.

TRAINER'S TIPS

Make sure only your forearms move during this exercise: the part of your arms from your elbows to your shoulders must remain still in order to properly stimulate the triceps.

LYING E–Z TRICEPS EXTENSION

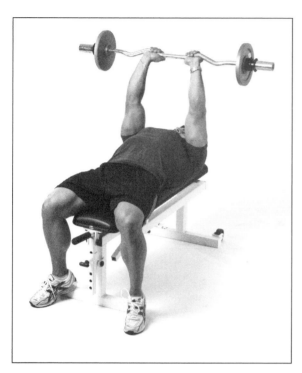

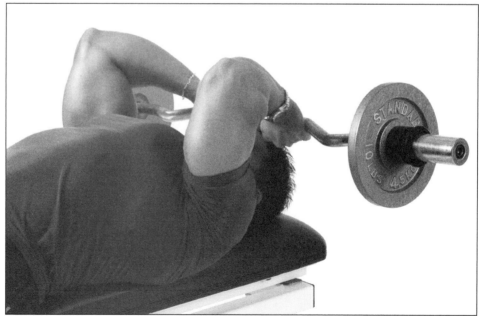

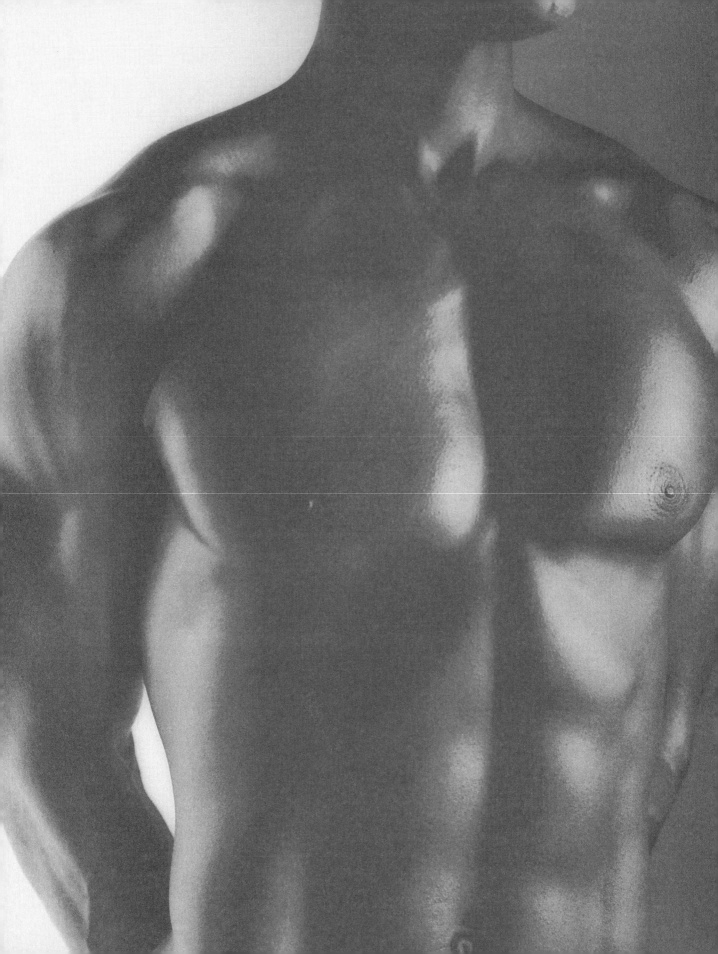

Chapter 7

The Core

Your core muscles are those at the center or trunk of your body—your abdominals, pelvis, back—which are essential for stabilization and work together to drive every movement you make. For every free–weight exercise you do, you need a strong center to execute the exercise in good form and safely.

The core exercises in this chapter make great use of the fitness ball. Training the core on the ball, a staple now in gyms which is easily purchasable, is an extremely efficient way to ensure that you target all the muscles of the core. When you perform an exercise on the ball, you recruit muscles in your back, your abdominals, and your pelvis, leaving your center stronger, sculpted, and powerful.

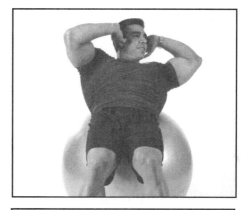

THE BODY SCULPTING BIBLE FOR
CHEST & ARMS

7

CRUNCH ON THE BALL

This variation of the traditional abdominal crunch allows for greater range of motion and increased recruitment of core stabilizers.

TECHNIQUE AND FORM

1 Sit on a fitness ball, then slide down until your lower back is on the ball. Your shoulders and upper back should be elevated.

2 Cross your arms behind your head and, as you exhale, slowly begin to lift your torso for three counts. Make sure your head is in line with your back (there should be ample space between your chin and chest).

3 At the same time that you lift your chest, lift one leg a few inches off the floor.

4 At the top position, hold for a count before lowering your torso and leg to the start position.

5 Repeat for the desired number of repetitions.

TRAINER'S TIPS

For a more intense balance and stabilization exercise, perform with one leg lifted and bent for the entire range of motion.

If you have trouble performing the exercise while lifting one leg, keep both in contact with the floor at all times.

Concentrate on keeping the ball as still as possible while performing the crunch.

If you do not have a ball, perform the same basic movement from the floor, (lifting your torso and then lowering).

CRUNCH ON THE BALL

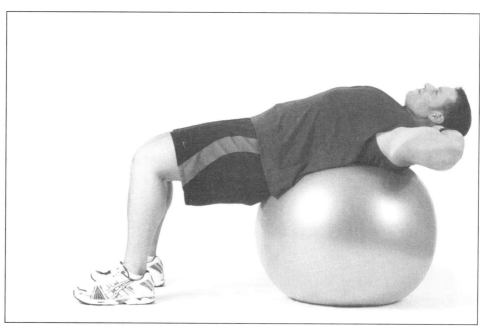

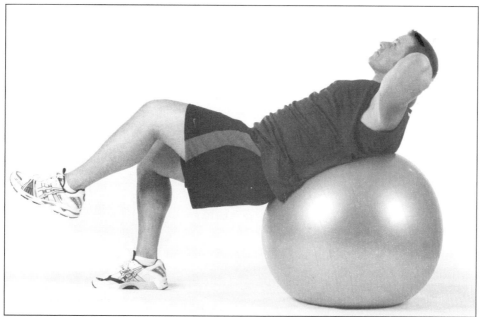

REVERSE CRUNCH WITH LEGS EXTENDED

Here's a great exercise for your overall core; if you are new to it, you may modify by keeping your legs bent.

TECHNIQUE AND FORM

1 Lie on the floor, grasping a fitness ball with your lower legs.

2 As you exhale, bring your legs up until they are perpendicular to the floor.

3 Slowly lower your legs until they are a few inches from the floor.

4 Hold for a count before repeating for desired number of repetitions.

TRAINER'S TIPS

◆ To relieve pressure on your lower back, place your hands beneath your back.

◆ If the exercise still strains your lower back, perform it with your knees bent instead of straight.

◆ Keep your head on the mat for the duration of this exercise.

◆ As you progress, when your legs reach the perpendicular position you can add a press up from your pelvis.

REVERSE CRUNCH WITH LEGS EXTENDED

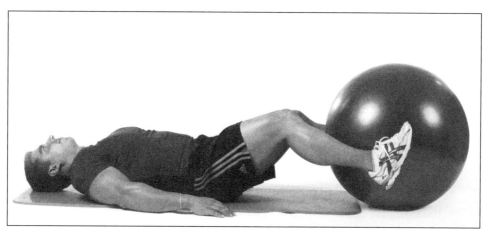

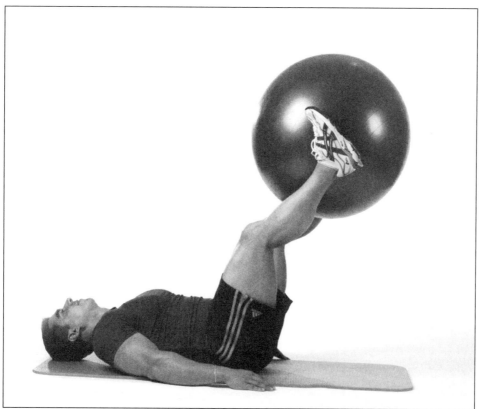

TWIST ON THE BALL

This is an exercise that maximizes recruitment of your obliques while also working the entire core. If you do not have a fitness ball, perform this exercise on a mat, keeping your shoulders elevated throughout the exercise as you twist from side to side.

TECHNIQUE AND FORM

1 Position yourself on the ball so that your lower back is supported. Your arms should be bent at the elbows and your head should be relaxed into the palms of your hands.

2 As you exhale, lift your chest and, leading with your right shoulder, twist over to your left knee.

3 Hold for a count until returning to the starting position.

4 Lift and twist, leading with your left shoulder, to your right knee.

5 Return to the start position.

6 Repeat for the desired number of repetitions, alternating the leading shoulder on each rep.

TRAINER'S TIPS

Make sure that you are leading with your shoulder and not pulling on your neck. Your chest should be open.

To increase the challenge of this exercise, lift your opposite leg off the ball as you perform the twist.

TWIST ON THE BALL

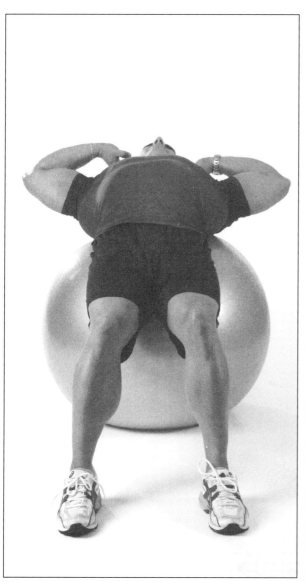
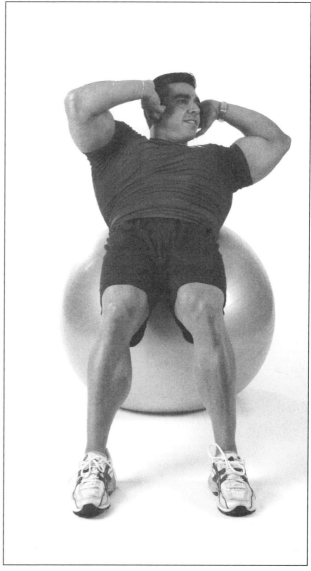

JACKKNIFE ON THE BALL

Here's an advanced exercise that requires upper body strength as well as a strong mid-section.

TECHNIQUE AND FORM

1 Get into a push–up position, with feet and lower legs resting on a fitness ball. Your hands should be on the floor, shoulder–width apart.

2 Pull your abs in as you bend your knees and bring your legs in to your chest. Your hips should lift to the ceiling. As you do this, exhale and curve your back to engage the abdominals.

3 Hold the top position for a count, before straightening back to the starting position.

4 Repeat for the desired number of repetitions.

TRAINER'S TIPS

✪ It is essential that you keep your abs pulled in and your glutes tight to keep your back flat (this avoids back strain.)

✪ To maximize muscle fiber recruitment, think about your abdominals as you pull the ball toward you.

✪ Release the contraction slowly, with control.

JACKKNIFE ON THE BALL

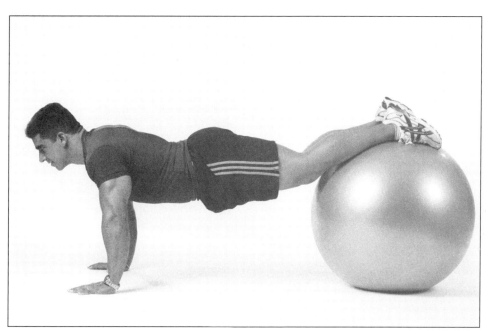

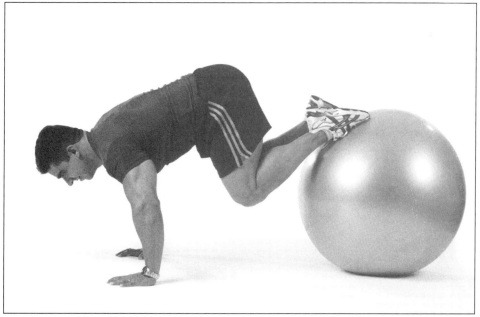

PLANK WITH ROTATION

A toughie, this exercise requires significant core (ab/back) strength. Work up to it.

TECHNIQUE AND FORM

1 Face the floor with your arms extended and shoulder–width apart, pull in your abdominals, and squeeze your glutes to keep your back flat. Hold that plank position for a couple of seconds.

2 Lift your right arm off the floor and rotate your body so that you are balancing on your left arm and left foot.

3 Rotate back and return your right hand to the floor.

4 Exhale and lift your left arm off the floor and rotate your body so that you are balancing on your right side.

5 Repeat for desired number of repetitions.

TRAINER'S TIPS

⊗ If the straight–arm plank is too difficult for you, you may perform this exercise with your forearms in contact with the floor.

⊗ Think about using your abs and lower back muscles to stabilize your body as you lift. Also think about grounding your body with the opposite arm and leg.

PLANK WITH ROTATION

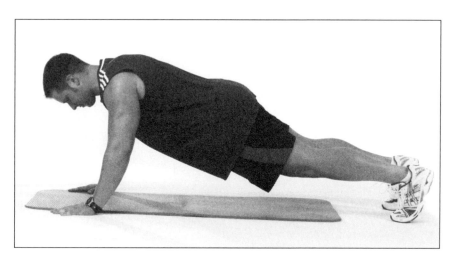

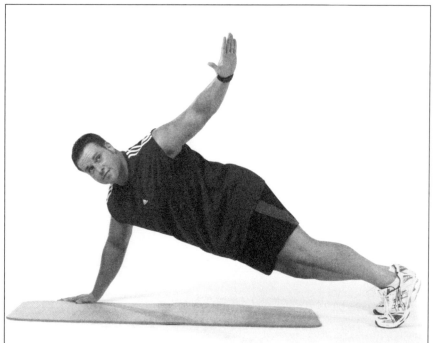

REVERSE CRUNCH

The reverse crunch targets the lower part of the abdominals.

TECHNIQUE AND FORM

1 Lie on a mat with your legs bent and raised from the floor.

2 Exhale and lift your hips slightly, bringing your knees in toward your chest. At the same time, lift your chest to meet your knees.

3 Hold the contraction for a second or two before releasing back to the start position.

4 Repeat for the desired number of repetitions.

TRAINER'S TIPS

Focus on pressing your belly button down into your spine at the same time as you lift your hips.

REVERSE CRUNCH

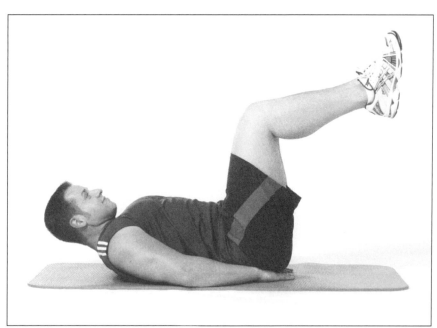

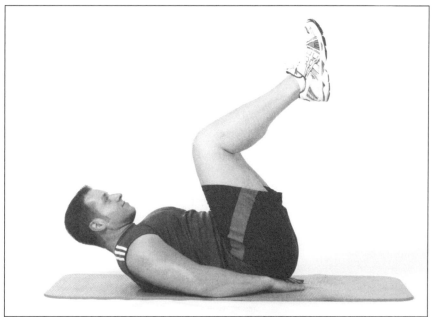

CRUNCH/PELVIC LIFT COMBINATION

This exercise targets both the outer and inner abdominals.

TECHNIQUE AND FORM

1 Lie on your back with your legs extended so that the soles of your feet face the ceiling. (Your legs should make a 90–degree angle with your body). Bend your arms behind your head.

2 As you exhale, slowly lift your torso, keeping your head in line with your spine.

3 At the same time, press your heels up to the ceiling by pressing your abs deep down through your spine.

4 Hold at the top position for a count or two before returning to a point where your shoulders don't quite touch the floor.

5 Repeat for the desired number of repetitions.

TRAINER'S TIPS

Make sure you keep your head back and that your neck is relaxed.

Try not to bring your shoulders down to the floor for the entire set. By keeping them slightly elevated you maintain tension and work in the muscles throughout the range of motion.

For the pelvic lift segment of the exercise it is important that you mentally focus on the lower part of your abdominals and that you minimize action in the hips. The movement is very small—your buttocks should rise just an inch or two from the floor.

CRUNCH/PELVIC LIFT COMBINATION

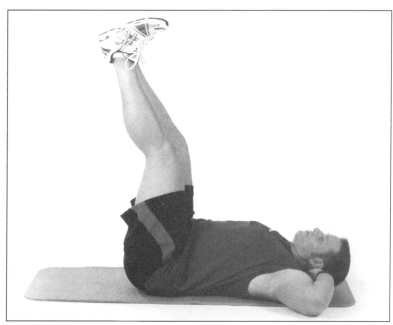

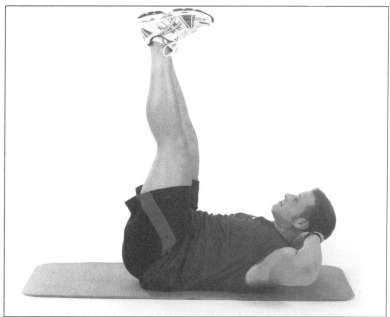

LOWER BACK EXTENSION

A great exercise to increase strength and support in your lower back; just be careful not to come up too high.

TECHNIQUE AND FORM

1 Lie on your stomach, with your legs extended and your head in line with your spine. Your arms should be straight down at your sides.

2 Exhale and slowly lift your torso and your legs simultaneously until you feel some pressure in your back.

3 Hold the top position for a couple of counts before returning to the starting position.

4 Repeat for the desired number of repetitions.

TRAINER'S TIPS

Be sure to lift only to the point of feeling some pressure in your lower back—if you feel any pain you are coming up too high and risking injury.

You can modify this exercise by lifting just the torso and keeping the legs in contact with the floor.

Another, more difficult variation is to perform this exercise with your arms extended over your head.

LOWER BACK EXTENSION

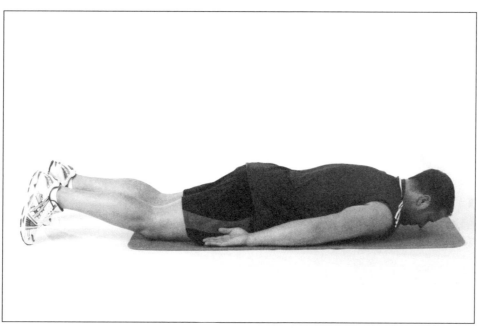

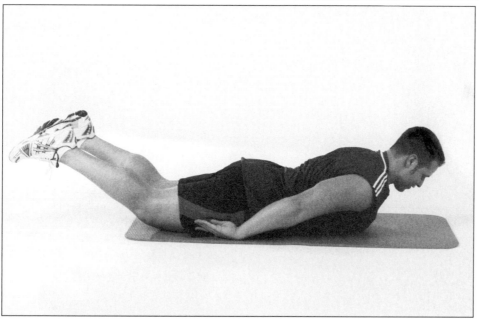

Part 3

The Workouts

Now you're ready to do the Chest & Arms Workout. The program offers three workouts, according to your level and goals: beginner, intermediate, and advanced. While primarily free–weight based, they also do include machine exercises. If you do not have access to machines, we indicate the free–weight alternatives for each machine exercise on the exercise description pages.

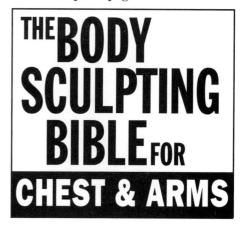

THE BODY SCULPTING BIBLE FOR CHEST & ARMS

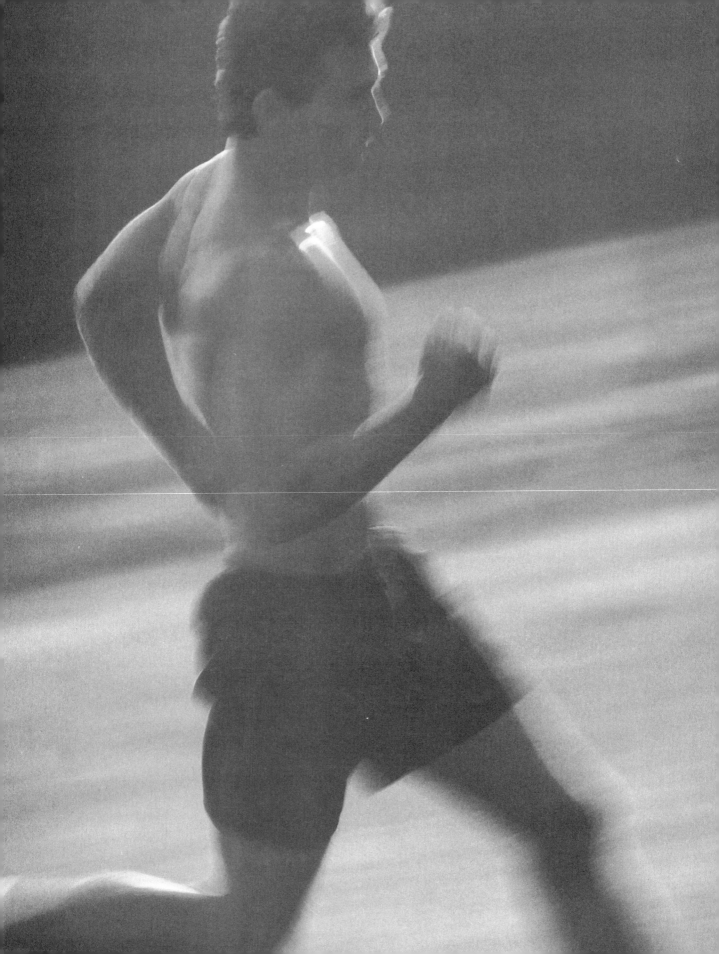

Chapter 8
Beginner Workout

The Beginner's workout involves performing exercises in pairs of modified compound supersets; working opposing muscle groups in each pair. Every two weeks, the program changes to ensure your muscles remain challenged.

Choose this workout program if you have been working out with weights for less than three months, or have taken time off. Check with your physician before beginning your exercise program.

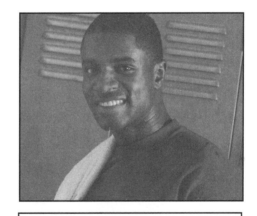

THE **BODY SCULPTING BIBLE** FOR

CHEST & ARMS

WEEKS 1 & 2

SPECIAL INSTRUCTIONS: Use pairs of modified compound supersets and perform 12–15 repetitions of each exercise and two sets.

DAY 1				MONDAY
EXERCISE	**PAGE NO.**	**REPS**	**SETS**	**REST**
MODIFIED COMPOUND SUPERSET # 1				
Back: Lat Pulldown (Wide Grip)	62	12–15	2	60 seconds
Chest: Incline Dumbbell Bench Press	46	12–15	2	60 seconds
MODIFIED COMPOUND SUPERSET # 2				
Back: One–Arm Row (Palms Facing Torso and Forward)	70	12–15	2	60 seconds
Chest: Dumbbell Fly	52	12–15	2	60 seconds
MODIFIED COMPOUND SUPERSET # 3				
Biceps: Hammer Curl with Rotation	96	12–15	2	60 seconds
Triceps: Overhead Dumbbell Triceps Extension	110	12–15	2	60 seconds
MODIFIED COMPOUND SUPERSET # 4				
Shoulders: Dumbbell Side Lateral	84	12–15	2	60 seconds
Shoulders: Rotator Cuff	90	12–15	2	60 seconds
ABS WORKOUT				
Crunch on the Ball	126	15	2	30 seconds
Reverse Crunch with Legs Extended	128	15	2	30 seconds
Twist on the Ball	130	15	2	30 seconds
Crunch/Pelvic Lift Combination	138	15	2	30 seconds
Lower Back Extension	140	15	2	30 seconds

Cardio: Perform 15 minutes of cardiovascular exercise such as elliptical training, stationary bike riding, running or jogging on a treadmill, or performing any other activity that will raise your heart rate to at least 220–(Your Age) x 0.75 +/– 10 beats.

DAY 2 — WEDNESDAY

EXERCISE	PAGE NO.	REPS	SETS	REST
ABS WORKOUT				
Crunch on the Ball	126	15	2	30 seconds
Reverse Crunch with Legs Extended	128	15	2	30 seconds
Twist on the Ball	130	15	2	30 seconds
Crunch/Pelvic Lift Combination	138	15	2	30 seconds
Lower Back Extension	140	15	2	30 seconds

Follow with a leg workout such as the one featured in *The Body Sculpting Bible for Men* (14–Day Body Sculpting Workout #1). Then perform 15 minutes of cardiovascular exercise such as elliptical training, stationary bike riding, running or jogging on a treadmill, or performing any other activity that will raise your heart rate to at least 220–(Your Age) x 0.75 +/– 10 beats.

DAY 3 — FRIDAY

EXERCISE	PAGE NO.	REPS	SETS	REST
MODIFIED COMPOUND SUPERSET # 1				
Back: Stiff Arm Pulldown	76	12–15	2	60 seconds
Chest: Incline Barbell Bench Press	46	12–15	2	60 seconds
MODIFIED COMPOUND SUPERSET # 2				
Back: Row Machine	64	12–15	2	60 seconds
Chest: Dumbbell Bench Press	48	12–15	2	60 seconds
MODIFIED COMPOUND SUPERSET # 3				
Biceps: High Cable Curl	100	12–15	2	60 seconds
Triceps: Triceps Dips	118	12–15	2	60 seconds
MODIFIED COMPOUND SUPERSET # 4				
Shoulders: Bent Over Lateral Raise	88	12–15	2	60 seconds
Shoulders: Military Press	86	12–15	2	60 seconds
ABS WORKOUT				
Crunch on the Ball	126	15	2	30 seconds
Reverse Crunch with Legs Extended	128	15	2	30 seconds
Twist on the Ball	130	15	2	30 seconds
Crunch/Pelvic Lift Combination	138	15	2	30 seconds
Lower Back Extension	140	15	2	30 seconds

Cardio: Perform 15 minutes of cardiovascular exercise such as elliptical training, stationary bike riding, running or jogging on a treadmill, or performing any other activity that will raise your heart rate to at least 220–(Your Age) x 0.75 +/– 10 beats.

WEEKS 3 & 4

SPECIAL INSTRUCTIONS: Use pairs of modified compound supersets and decrease rest period to 45 seconds. In addition, add another pair of arm exercises to the routine.

DAY 1				MONDAY
EXERCISE	**PAGE NO.**	**REPS**	**SETS**	**REST**
MODIFIED COMPOUND SUPERSET # 1				
Back: Lat Pulldown (Wide Grip)	62	12–15	2	45 seconds
Chest: Incline Dumbbell Bench Press	46	12–15	2	45 seconds
MODIFIED COMPOUND SUPERSET # 2				
Back: One–Arm Row (Palms Facing Torso and Forward)	70	12–15	2	45 seconds
Chest: Dumbbell Fly	52	12–15	2	45 seconds
MODIFIED COMPOUND SUPERSET # 3				
Biceps: Hammer Curl with Rotation	96	12–15	2	45 seconds
Triceps: Overhead Dumbbell Triceps Extension	110	12–15	2	45 seconds
MODIFIED COMPOUND SUPERSET # 4				
Biceps: Curl (Arms Turned Out)	102	12–15	2	45 seconds
Triceps: Triceps Pushdown (bar)	84	12–15	2	45 seconds
MODIFIED COMPOUND SUPERSET # 5				
Shoulders: Dumbbell Side Lateral	90	12–15	2	45 seconds
Shoulders: Rotator Cuff	84	12–15	2	45 seconds
ABS WORKOUT				
Crunch on the Ball	90	15	2	30 seconds
Reverse Crunch with Legs Extended	126	15	2	30 seconds
Twist on the Ball	130	15	2	30 seconds
Crunch/Pelvic Lift Combination	138	15	2	30 seconds
Lower Back Extension	140	15	2	30 seconds

Cardio: Perform 15 minutes of cardiovascular exercise such as elliptical training, stationary bike riding, running or jogging on a treadmill, or performing any other activity that will raise your heart rate to at least 220–(Your Age) x 0.75 +/− 10 beats.

DAY 2				WEDNESDAY
EXERCISE	**PAGE NO.**	**REPS**	**SETS**	**REST**
ABS WORKOUT				
Crunch on the Ball	126	15	2	30 seconds
Reverse Crunch with Legs Extended	128	15	2	30 seconds
Twist on the Ball	130	15	2	30 seconds
Crunch/Pelvic Lift Combination	138	15	2	30 seconds
Lower Back Extension	140	15	2	30 seconds

Follow with a leg workout such as the one featured in *The Body Sculpting Bible for Men* (14–Day Body Sculpting Workout #1). Then perform 15 minutes of cardiovascular exercise such as elliptical training, stationary bike riding, running or jogging on a treadmill, or performing any other activity that will raise your heart rate to at least 220–(Your Age) x 0.75 +/– 10 beats.

DAY 3				FRIDAY
EXERCISE	**PAGE NO.**	**REPS**	**SETS**	**REST**
MODIFIED COMPOUND SUPERSET # 1				
Back: Stiff Arm Pulldown	76	12–15	2	45 seconds
Chest: Incline Barbell Bench Press	46	12–15	2	45 seconds
MODIFIED COMPOUND SUPERSET # 2				
Back: Row Machine	64	12–15	2	45 seconds
Chest: Dumbbell Bench Press	48	12–15	2	45 seconds
MODIFIED COMPOUND SUPERSET # 3				
Biceps: Preacher Curl	108	12–15	2	45 seconds
Triceps: Triceps Pushdown (rope)	114	12–15	2	45 seconds
MODIFIED COMPOUND SUPERSET # 4				
Biceps: High Cable Curl	100	12–15	2	45 seconds
Triceps: Triceps Dip	118	12–15	2	45 seconds
MODIFIED COMPOUND SUPERSET # 5				
Shoulders: Bent Over Lateral Raise	88	12–15	2	45 seconds
Shoulders: Military Press	86	12–15	2	45 seconds

Cardio: Perform 15 minutes of cardiovascular exercise such as elliptical training, stationary bike riding, running or jogging on a treadmill, or performing any other activity that will raise your heart rate to at least 220–(Your Age) x 0.75 +/– 10 beats.

WEEKS 5 & 6

SPECIAL INSTRUCTIONS: Use pairs of modified compound supersets. Performing 10 to 12 reps in each set, increase to three sets per exercise.

DAY 1				MONDAY
EXERCISE	**PAGE NO.**	**REPS**	**SETS**	**REST**
MODIFIED COMPOUND SUPERSET # 1				
Back: Lat Pulldown (Wide Grip)	62	10–12	3	45 seconds
Chest: Incline Dumbbell Bench Press	46	10–12	3	45 seconds
MODIFIED COMPOUND SUPERSET # 2				
Back: One-Arm Row (Palms Facing Torso and Forward)	70	10–12	3	45 seconds
Chest: Dumbbell Fly	52	10–12	3	45 seconds
MODIFIED COMPOUND SUPERSET # 3				
Biceps: Hammer Curl with Rotation	96	10–12	3	45 seconds
Triceps: Overhead Dumbbell Triceps Extension	110	10–12	3	45 seconds
MODIFIED COMPOUND SUPERSET # 4				
Biceps: Curl (Arms Turned Out)	102	10–12	3	45 seconds
Triceps: Triceps Pushdown (bar)	114	10–12	3	45 seconds
MODIFIED COMPOUND SUPERSET # 5				
Shoulders: Dumbbell Side Lateral	84	10–12	3	45 seconds
Shoulders: Rotator Cuff	90	10–12	3	45 seconds
ABS WORKOUT				
Crunch on the Ball	126	15	2	30 seconds
Reverse Crunch with Legs Extended	128	15	2	30 seconds
Twist on the Ball	130	15	2	30 seconds
Crunch/Pelvic Lift Combination	138	15	2	30 seconds
Lower Back Extension	140	15	2	30 seconds

Cardio: Perform 20 minutes of cardiovascular exercise such as elliptical training, stationary bike riding, running or jogging on a treadmill, or performing any other activity that will raise your heart rate to at least 220–(Your Age) x 0.75 +/– 10 beats.

DAY 2 — WEDNESDAY

EXERCISE	PAGE NO.	REPS	SETS	REST
ABS WORKOUT				
Crunch on the Ball	126	15	2	30 seconds
Reverse Crunch with Legs Extended	128	15	2	30 seconds
Twist on the Ball	130	15	2	30 seconds
Crunch/Pelvic Lift Combination	138	15	2	30 seconds
Lower Back Extension	140	15	2	30 seconds

Follow with a leg workout such as the one featured in *The Body Sculpting Bible for Men* (14–Day Body Sculpting Workout #1). Then perform 20 minutes of cardiovascular exercise such as elliptical training, stationary bike riding, running or jogging on a treadmill, or performing any other activity that will raise your heart rate to at least 220–(Your Age) x 0.75 +/– 10 beats.

DAY 3 — FRIDAY

EXERCISE	PAGE NO.	REPS	SETS	REST
MODIFIED COMPOUND SUPERSET # 1				
Back: Stiff Arm Pulldown	76	10–12	3	45 seconds
Chest: Incline Barbell Bench Press	46	10–12	3	45 seconds
MODIFIED COMPOUND SUPERSET # 2				
Back: Row Machine	64	10–12	3	45 seconds
Chest: Dumbbell Bench Press	48	10–12	3	45 seconds
MODIFIED COMPOUND SUPERSET # 3				
Biceps: Preacher Curl	108	10–12	3	45 seconds
Triceps: Triceps Pushdown (rope)	114	10–12	3	45 seconds
MODIFIED COMPOUND SUPERSET # 4				
Biceps: High Cable Curl	100	10–12	3	45 seconds
Triceps: Triceps Dip	118	10–12	3	45 seconds
MODIFIED COMPOUND SUPERSET # 5				
Shoulders: Bent Over Lateral Raise	88	10–12	3	45 seconds
Shoulders: Military Press	86	10–12	3	45 seconds
ABS WORKOUT				
Crunch on the Ball	126	15	2	30 seconds
Reverse Crunch with Legs Extended	128	15	2	30 seconds
Twist on the Ball	130	15	2	30 seconds
Crunch/Pelvic Lift Combination	138	15	2	30 seconds
Lower Back Extension	140	15	2	30 seconds

Cardio: Perform 20 minutes of cardiovascular exercise such as elliptical training, stationary bike riding, running or jogging on a treadmill, or performing any other activity that will raise your heart rate to at least 220–(Your Age) x 0.75 +/– 10 beats.

WEEKS 7 & 8

SPECIAL INSTRUCTIONS: Use pairs of supersets. Remove rest in between exercises in each set.

DAY 1				MONDAY
EXERCISE	**PAGE NO.**	**REPS**	**SETS**	**REST**
SUPERSET # 1				
Back: Lat Pulldown (Wide Grip)	62	10–12	3	0 seconds
Chest: Incline Dumbbell Bench Press	46	10–12	3	45 seconds
SUPERSET # 2				
Back: One-Arm Rows (Palms Facing Torso and Forward)	70	10–12	3	0 seconds
Chest: Dumbbell Fly	52	10–12	3	45 seconds
SUPERSET # 3				
Biceps: Hammer Curl with Rotation	96	10–12	3	0 seconds
Triceps: Overhead Dumbbell Triceps Extension	110	10–12	3	45 seconds
SUPERSET # 4				
Biceps: Curl (Arms Turned Out)	102	10–12	3	0 seconds
Triceps: Triceps Pushdown (bar)	84	10–12	3	45 seconds
SUPERSET # 5				
Shoulders: Dumbbell Side Lateral	90	10–12	3	0 seconds
Shoulders: Rotator Cuff	84	10–12	3	45 seconds
ABS WORKOUT				
Crunch on the Ball	90	15	2	30 seconds
Reverse Crunch with Legs Extended	126	15	2	30 seconds
Twist on the Ball	130	15	2	30 seconds
Crunch/Pelvic Lift Combination	138	15	2	30 seconds
Lower Back Extension	140	15	2	30 seconds

Cardio: Perform 20 minutes of cardiovascular exercise such as elliptical training, stationary bike riding, running or jogging on a treadmill, or performing any other activity that will raise your heart rate to at least 220–(Your Age) x 0.75 +/– 10 beats.

DAY 2 — WEDNESDAY

EXERCISE	PAGE NO.	REPS	SETS	REST
ABS WORKOUT				
Crunch on the Ball	126	15	2	30 seconds
Reverse Crunch with Legs Extended	128	15	2	30 seconds
Twist on the Ball	130	15	2	30 seconds
Crunch/Pelvic Lift Combination	138	15	2	30 seconds
Lower Back Extension	140	15	2	30 seconds

Follow with a leg workout such as the one featured in *The Body Sculpting Bible for Men* (14–Day Body Sculpting Workout #1). Then perform 20 minutes of cardiovascular exercise such as elliptical training, stationary bike riding, running or jogging on a treadmill, or performing any other activity that will raise your heart rate to at least 220–(Your Age) x 0.75 +/– 10 beats.

DAY 3 — FRIDAY

EXERCISE	PAGE NO.	REPS	SETS	REST
MODIFIED COMPOUND SUPERSET # 1				
Back: Stiff Arm Pulldown	76	10–12	3	0 seconds
Chest: Incline Barbell Bench Press	46	10–12	3	45 seconds
MODIFIED COMPOUND SUPERSET # 2				
Back: Row Machine	64	10–12	3	0 seconds
Chest: Dumbbell Bench Press	48	10–12	3	45 seconds
MODIFIED COMPOUND SUPERSET # 3				
Biceps: Preacher Curl	108	10–12	3	0 seconds
Triceps: Triceps Pushdown (rope)	114	10–12	3	45 seconds
MODIFIED COMPOUND SUPERSET # 4				
Biceps: High Cable Curl	100	10–12	3	0 seconds
Triceps: Triceps Dip	118	10–12	3	45 seconds
MODIFIED COMPOUND SUPERSET # 5				
Shoulders: Bent Over Lateral Raise	88	10–12	3	0 seconds
Shoulders: Military Press	86	10–12	3	45 seconds
ABS WORKOUT				
Crunch on the Ball	90	15	2	30 seconds
Reverse Crunch with Legs Extended	126	15	2	30 seconds
Twist on the Ball	130	15	2	30 seconds
Crunch/Pelvic Lift Combination	138	15	2	30 seconds
Lower Back Extension	140	15	2	30 seconds

Cardio: Perform 20 minutes of cardiovascular exercise such as elliptical training, stationary bike riding, running or jogging on a treadmill, or performing any other activity that will raise your heart rate to at least 220–(Your Age) x 0.75 +/– 10 beats.

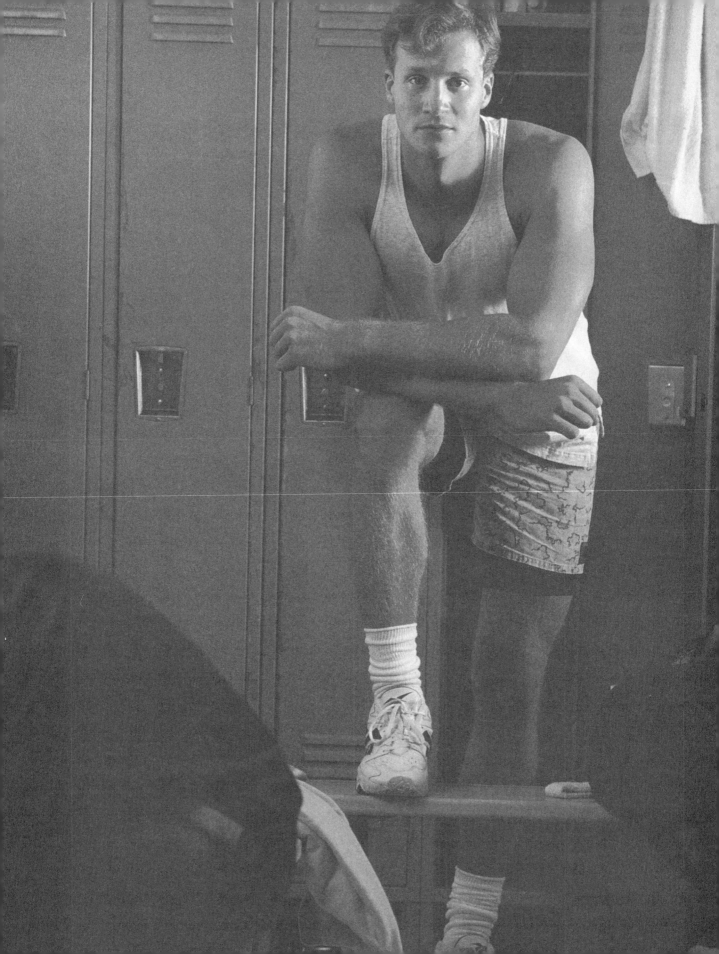

Chapter 9
Intermediate Workout

The Intermediate program involves compound supersets composed of consecutive exercises for a single muscle group. Since this workout emphasizes muscle definition, we grouped exercises for the same muscle group together.

Choose the Intermediate Workout if you have been training for three months to one year.

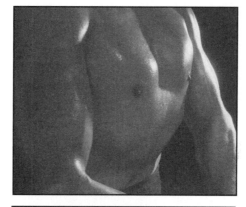

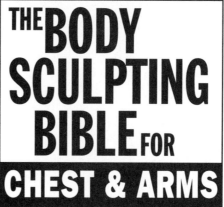

THE BODY SCULPTING BIBLE FOR CHEST & ARMS

9

WEEKS 1 & 2

SPECIAL INSTRUCTIONS:

- Perform 12 to15 repetitions of each exercise and two sets.
- Note that the pace of the workout is fast as well in order to emphasize definition.
- In many cases we provide a couple of exercise choices. In order to incorporate variety in your workouts, it is recommended that one day you choose one exercise and then the next training session you perform the other one.

DAY 1 AND 4				MONDAY AND THURSDAY
EXERCISE	**PAGE NO.**	**REPS**	**SETS**	**REST**
MODIFIED COMPOUND SUPERSET # 1				
Back: Lat Pulldown or Pull-Up (Wide Grip) (May use Pull–Up Assist Machine)	62 or 72	12–15	2	30 seconds
Back: Pull-Up (Reverse Grip)	74	12–15	2	30 seconds
Back: One-Arm Row (Palms Facing Torso and Forward) or Low Pulley Cable Row	70 or 68	12–15	2	30 seconds
Back: Stiff Arm Pulldowns	76	12–15	2	60 seconds
MODIFIED COMPOUND SUPERSET # 2				
Chest: Incline Barbell Bench Press	46	12–15	2	30 seconds
Chest: Incline Dumbbell Bench Press	46	12–15	2	30 seconds
Chest: Dumbbell Bench Press or Chest Dip	48 or 58	12–15	2	30 seconds
Chest: Dumbbell Incline Fly or Incline Cable Fly	50 or 54	12–15	2	60 seconds
ABS WORKOUT				
Crunch on the Ball	126	30	2	30 seconds
Reverse Crunch with Legs Extended	128	30	2	30 seconds
Twist on the Ball	130	30	2	30 seconds
Crunch/Pelvic Lift Combination	138	30	2	30 seconds
Reverse Crunch	136	30	2	30 seconds
Lower Back Extension	140	30	2	30 seconds

Cardio: Perform 20 minutes of cardiovascular exercise such as elliptical training, stationary bike riding, running or jogging on a treadmill, or performing any other activity that will raise your heart rate to at least 220–(Your Age) x 0.75 +/– 10 beats.

WEEKS 1 & 2

DAY 2 AND 5 — TUESDAY AND FRIDAY

EXERCISE	PAGE NO.	REPS	SETS	REST
MODIFIED COMPOUND SUPERSET # 1				
Biceps: Preacher Curl or Alternate Dumbbell Curl	108 or 94	12–15	2	30 seconds
Biceps: Concentration Curl or Preacher Curl	104 or 108	12–15	2	30 seconds
Biceps: Hammer Curl with Rotation or Incline Hammer Curl	96 or 98	12–15	2	30 seconds
Biceps: Incline Curl	100	12–15	2	60 seconds
MODIFIED COMPOUND SUPERSET # 2				
Triceps: Triceps Pushdown	115	12–15	2	30 seconds
Triceps: Overhead Dumbbell Triceps Extension	110	12–15	2	30 seconds
Triceps: Kickback or Lying Triceps Extension	113 or 120	12–15	2	30 seconds
Triceps: Close Grip Bench Press or Triceps Dip	116 or 118	12–15	2	60 seconds
MODIFIED COMPOUND SUPERSET # 3				
Shoulders: Military Press or Upright Row	86 or 80	12–15	2	30 seconds
Shoulders: Dumbbell Side Lateral	84	12–15	2	30 seconds
Shoulders: Rotator Cuff	90	12–15	2	30 seconds
Shoulders: Rear Delt on Machine or Bent-Over Lateral Raise	78 or 88	12–15	2	60 seconds

Cardio: Perform 20 minutes of cardiovascular exercise such as elliptical training, stationary bike riding, running or jogging on a treadmill, or performing any other activity that will raise your heart rate to at least 220–(Your Age) x 0.75 +/– 10 beats.

DAY 3 AND 6 — WEDNESDAY AND SATURDAY

On Wednesdays and Saturdays you can perform the leg workout portion from the Advanced 14–Day Body Sculpting Program presented in *The Body Sculpting Bible for Men* followed by 20 minutes of cardiovascular exercise such as elliptical training, biking,running or jogging on a treadmill, or performing any other activity that will raise your heart rate to at least 220–(Your Age) x 0.75 +/– 10 beats.

WEEKS 3 & 4

SPECIAL INSTRUCTIONS:

- Perform 10–12 repetitions of each exercise and three sets.
- Eliminate the rest in between some of the exercises as prescribed.
- In many cases we provide a couple of exercises choices. In order to incorporate variety in your workouts, it is recommended that one day you choose one exercise and then the next training session you perform the other one.

DAY 1 AND 4				MONDAY AND THURSDAY
EXERCISE	**PAGE NO.**	**REPS**	**SETS**	**REST**
SUPERSET # 1				
Back: Lat Pulldown or Pull-Up (Wide Grip) (May use Pull–Up Assist Machine)	62 or 72	10–12	3	0 seconds
Back: Pull–Up (Reverse Grip) or Low Pulley Cable Row	74 or 68	10–12	3	30 seconds
Back: One-Arm Row (Palms Facing Torso and Forward) or Low Pulley Cable Row	70 or 68	10–12	3	0 seconds
Back: Stiff Arm Pulldown	76	10–12	3	60 seconds
SUPERSET # 2				
Chest: Incline Barbell Bench Press	46	10–12	3	0 seconds
Chest: Incline Dumbbell Bench Press	46	10–12	3	30 seconds
Chest: Dumbbell Bench Press or Chest Dip	48	10–12	3	0 seconds
Chest: Dumbbell Incline Fly or Incline Cable Fly	50 or 54	10–12	3	60 seconds
ABS WORKOUT				
Crunch on the Ball	126	30	3	30 seconds
Reverse Crunch with Legs Extended	128	30	3	30 seconds
Twist on the Ball	130	30	3	30 seconds
Crunch/Pelvic Lift Combination	138	30	3	30 seconds
Reverse Crunch	136	30	3	30 seconds
Lower Back Extension	140	30	3	30 seconds
Cardio: Perform 30 minutes of cardiovascular exercise such as elliptical training, stationary bike riding, running or jogging on a treadmill, or performing any other activity that will raise your heart rate to at least 220–(Your Age) x 0.75 +/– 10 beats.				

WEEKS 3 & 4

DAY 2 AND 5				TUESDAY AND FRIDAY
EXERCISE	**PAGE NO.**	**REPS**	**SETS**	**REST**
SUPERSET # 1				
Biceps: Preacher Curl or Alternate Dumbbell Curl	108 or 94	10–12	3	0 seconds
Biceps: Concentration Curl or Preacher Curl	104 or 108	10–12	3	30 seconds
Biceps: Hammer Curl with Rotation or Incline Hammer Curl	96 or 98	10–12	3	0 seconds
Biceps: Incline Curl	100	10–12	3	60 seconds
SUPERSET # 2				
Triceps: Triceps Pushdown	114	10–12	3	0 seconds
Triceps: Overhead Dumbbell Triceps Extension	110	10–12	3	30 seconds
Triceps: Kickback or Lying Triceps Extension	112 or 120	10–12	3	0 seconds
Triceps: Close Grip Bench Press or Triceps Dip	116 or 118	10–12	3	60 seconds
SUPERSET # 3				
Shoulders: Military Press or Upright Row	86 or 80	10–12	3	0 seconds
Shoulders: Dumbbell Side Lateral	84	10–12	3	30 seconds
Shoulders: Rotator Cuff	90	10–12	3	0 seconds
Shoulders: Rear Delt on Machine or Bent-Over Lateral Raise	78 or 88	10–12	3	60 seconds

Cardio: Perform 30 minutes of cardiovascular exercise such as elliptical training, stationary bike riding, running or jogging on a treadmill, or performing any other activity that will raise your heart rate to at least 220–(Your Age) x 0.75 +/– 10 beats.

DAY 3 AND 6	WEDNESDAY AND SATURDAY

On Wednesdays and Saturdays you can perform the leg workout portion from the Advanced 14–Day Body Sculpting Program presented in *The Body Sculpting Bible for Men* followed by 30 minutes of cardiovascular exercise such as elliptical training, biking,running or jogging on a treadmill, or performing any other activity that will raise your heart rate to at least 220–(Your Age) x 0.75 +/– 10 beats.

WEEKS 5 & 6

SPECIAL INSTRUCTIONS:

- Perform 8 to 10 repetitions and three or four sets for each exercise as described.
- Perform the exercises as giant sets.
- In many cases we provide a couple of exercises choices. In order to incorporate variety in your workouts, it is recommended that one day you choose one exercise and then the next training session you perform the other one.

DAY 1 AND 4				MONDAY AND THURSDAY
EXERCISE	**PAGE NO.**	**REPS**	**SETS**	**REST**
GIANT SET # 1				
Back: Lat Pulldown or Pull-Up (Wide Grip) (May use Pull–Up Assist Machine)	62 or 72	8–10	4	0 seconds
Back: Pull–ups (Reverse Grip) or Low Pulley Cable Row	74 or 68	8–10	4	0 seconds
Back: One-Arm Row (Palms Facing Torso and Forward) or Low Pulley Cable Rows	70 or 68	8–10	4	0 seconds
Back: Stiff Arm Pulldown	76	8–10	4	60 seconds
GIANT SET # 2				
Chest: Incline Barbell Bench Press	46	8–10	4	0 seconds
Chest: Incline Dumbbell Bench Press	46	8–10	4	0 seconds
Chest: Dumbbell Bench Press or Chest Dip	48	8–10	4	0 seconds
Chest: Dumbbell Incline Fly or Incline Cable Fly	50 or 54	8–10	4	60 seconds
ABS WORKOUT				
Crunch on the Ball	126	30	3	30 seconds
Reverse Crunch with Legs Extended	128	30	3	30 seconds
Twist on the Ball	130	30	3	30 seconds
Crunch/Pelvic Lift Combination	138	30	3	30 seconds
Reverse Crunch	136	30	3	30 seconds
Lower Back Extension	140	30	3	30 seconds
Cardio: Perform 40 minutes of cardiovascular exercise such as elliptical training, stationary bike riding, running or jogging on a treadmill, or performing any other activity that will raise your heart rate to at least 220–(Your Age) x 0.75 +/– 10 beats.				

WEEKS 5 & 6

EXERCISE	PAGE NO.	REPS	SETS	REST
GIANT SET # 1				
Biceps: Preacher Curl or Alternate Dumbbell Curl	108 or 94	8–10	3	0 seconds
Biceps: Concentration Curl or Preacher Curl	104 or 108	8–10	3	0 seconds
Biceps: Hammer Curl with Rotation or Incline Hammer Curls	96 or 98	8–10	3	0 seconds
Biceps: Incline Curl	100	8–10	3	60 seconds
GIANT SET # 2				
Triceps: Triceps Pushdown	114	8–10	3	0 seconds
Triceps: Overhead Dumbbell Triceps Extension	110	8–10	3	0 seconds
Triceps: Kickback or Lying Triceps Extension	112 or 120	8–10	3	0 seconds
Triceps: Close Grip Bench Press or Triceps Dip	116 or 118	8–10	3	60 seconds
GIANT SET # 3				
Shoulders: Military Press or Upright Row	86 or 80	8–10	3	0 seconds
Shoulders: Dumbbell Side Lateral	84	8–10	3	0 seconds
Shoulders: Rotator Cuff	90	8–10	3	0 seconds
Shoulders: Rear Delt on Machine or Bent-Over Lateral Raise	78 or 88	8–10	3	60 seconds

Cardio: Perform 40 minutes of cardiovascular exercise such as elliptical training, stationary bike riding, running or jogging on a treadmill, or performing any other activity that will raise your heart rate to at least 220–(Your Age) x 0.75 +/– 10 beats.

On Wednesdays and Saturdays you can perform the leg workout portion from the Advanced 14–Day Body Sculpting Program presented in *The Body Sculpting Bible for Men* followed by 40 minutes of cardiovascular exercise such as elliptical training, biking, running or jogging on a treadmill, or performing any other activity that will raise your heart rate to at least 220–(Your Age) x 0.75 +/– 10 beats.

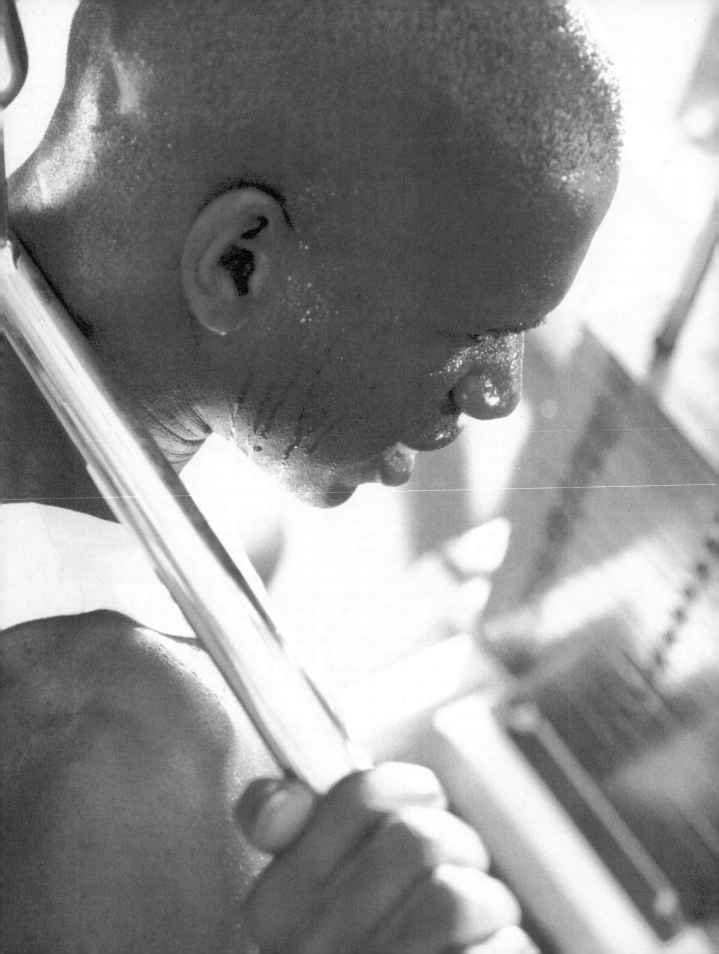

Chapter 10
Advanced Workout

Choose the Advanced Workout if you have been exercising for at least one year and want to build muscle mass.

The Advanced program involves compound supersets composed of consecutive exercises for two opposing muscle groups. Since this workout emphasizes building muscle mass, we grouped exercises for opposite muscle groups together.

The pace of the workout is a bit slower and the repetition ranges are lower in order to emphasize muscle mass. In addition, the exercises selected are exercises that recruit the most muscle fibers in order to get the fastest muscle mass gains in the shortest amount of time.

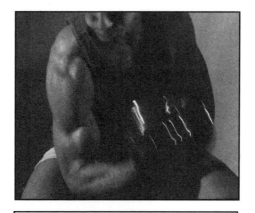

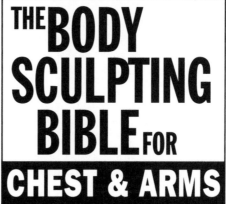

THE BODY SCULPTING BIBLE FOR CHEST & ARMS

10

WEEKS 1 & 2

SPECIAL INSTRUCTIONS:

- Perform 10–12 repetitions of each exercise and two or three sets.
- Each exercise includes an alternate choice. The alternate is to be performed the second time that you hit the same muscle group on that week. This is crucial in order to keep the body off balance and thus continue to trigger muscle mass gains.

DAY 1 AND 4				MONDAY AND THURSDAY
EXERCISE	**PAGE NO.**	**REPS**	**SETS**	**REST**
MODIFIED COMPOUND SUPERSET # 1				
Back: Pull–Up (Wide Grip) (alternate: Pull–Up (Close Grip)	72	10–12	3	60 seconds
Chest: Incline Dumbbell Bench Press (alternate: Incline Barbell Bench Press)	46	10–12	3	60 seconds
Back: Pull–Up (Reverse Grip) (alternate: Pull–Up (Medium Grip))	74 or 72	10–12	3	60 seconds
Chest: Chest Dip (alternate: Incline Dumbbell Bench Press)	58 or 46	10–12	3	60 seconds
MODIFIED COMPOUND SUPERSET # 2				
Chest: Barbell Bench Press (alternate: Dumbbell Bench Press)	46	10–12	3	60 seconds
Back: Row Machine (alternate: One-Arm Row)	64 or 70	10–12	3	60 seconds
Chest: Incline Cable Fly (alternate: Pullover)	52 or 66	10–12	3	60 seconds
Back: Stiff Arm Pulldown (bar) (alternate: Stiff Arm Pulldown (rope)	76	10–12	3	60 seconds
ABS WORKOUT				
Crunch on the Ball	126	20	2	15 seconds
Reverse Crunch with Legs Extended	128	20	2	15 seconds
Twist on the Ball	130	20	2	15 seconds
Crunch/Pelvic Lift Combination	138	20	2	15 seconds
Reverse Crunch	136	20	2	15 seconds
Plank with Rotation	134	20	2	15 seconds
Lower Back Extension	140	20	2	15 seconds

DAY 2 AND 5 — TUESDAY AND FRIDAY

EXERCISE	PAGE NO.	REPS	SETS	REST
MODIFIED COMPOUND SUPERSET # 1				
Biceps: Preacher Curl (alternate: Concentration Curl)	108 or 104	10–12	3	60 seconds
Triceps: Triceps Dip (alternate: Lying Triceps Extension)	118 or 120	10–12	3	60 seconds
Biceps: Hammer Curl with Rotation (alternate: Reverse E-Z Curl)	96 or 106	10–12	2	60 seconds
Triceps: Triceps Pushdown (rope) (alternate: Triceps Pushdown (bar))	114	10–12	2	60 seconds
MODIFIED COMPOUND SUPERSET # 2				
Biceps: High Cable Curl (alternate: Reverse E-Z Curl)	100 or 106	10–12	3	60 seconds
Triceps: Close Grip Bench Press (alternate: Overhead Dumbbell Triceps Extension)	116 or 110	10–12	3	60 seconds
Biceps: Dumbbell Curl (alternate: High Cable Curl)	94 or 100	10–12	2	60 seconds
Triceps: Lying E-Z Triceps Extension (alternate: Triceps Dip)	122 or 118	10–12	2	60 seconds
MODIFIED COMPOUND SUPERSET # 3				
Shoulders: Bent-Over Lateral Raise (alternate: Rear Delt on Machine)	88 or 78	10–12	3	60 seconds
Shoulders: Rotator Cuff	90	10–12	3	60 seconds
Shoulders: Cable Lateral (alternate: Dumbbell Side Lateral)	82 or 84	10–12	3	60 seconds
Shoulders: Upright Row (alternate: Military Press)	80 or 86	10–12	3	60 seconds

DAY 3 AND 6 — WEDNESDAY AND SATURDAY

On Wednesdays and Saturdays you can perform the leg workout portion from the Advanced 14–Day Body Sculpting Program presented in *The Body Sculpting Bible for Men* followed by 20 minutes of cardiovascular exercise such as elliptical training, biking, running or jogging on a treadmill, or performing any other activity that will raise your heart rate to at least 220–(Your Age) x 0.75 +/– 10 beats.

WEEKS 3 & 4

SPECIAL INSTRUCTIONS:

- Perform 8–10 repetitions of each exercise for two, three or four sets as noted below.
- Eliminate the rest in between some of the exercises as prescribed below.
- Each exercise includes an alternate choice. The alternate is to be performed on the second time that you hit the same muscle group on that week. This is crucial in order to keep the body off balance and thus continue to trigger muscle mass gains.

DAY 1 AND 4				MONDAY AND THURSDAY
EXERCISE	**PAGE NO.**	**REPS**	**SETS**	**REST**
SUPERSET # 1				
Back: Pull–Up (Wide Grip) (alternate: Pull–Up (Close Grip)	72	8–10	4	0 seconds
Chest: Incline Dumbbell Bench Press (alternate: Incline Barbell Bench Press)	46	8–10	4	60 seconds
Back: Pull–Up (Reverse Grip) (alternate: Pull–Up (Medium Grip))	74 or 72	8–10	3	0 seconds
Chest: Chest Dip (alternate: Incline Dumbbell Bench Press)	58 or 46	8–10	3	60 seconds
SUPERSET # 2				
Chest: Barbell Bench Press (alternate: Dumbbell Bench Press)	48	8–10	4	0 seconds
Back: Row Machine (alternate: One-Arm Row)	64 or 70	8–10	4	60 seconds
Chest: Incline Cable Fly (alternate: Pullover)	52 or 66	8–10	3	0 seconds
Back: Stiff Arm Pulldown (bar) (alternate: Stiff Arm Pulldown (rope)	76	8–10	3	60 seconds
ABS WORKOUT				
Crunch on the Ball	126	20	3	15 seconds
Reverse Crunch with Legs Extended	128	20	3	15 seconds
Twist on the Ball	130	20	3	15 seconds
Crunch/Pelvic Lift Combination	138	20	3	15 seconds
Reverse Crunch	136	20	3	15 seconds
Plank with Rotation	134	20	3	15 seconds
Lower Back Extension	140	20	3	15 seconds

DAY 2 AND 5				TUESDAY AND FRIDAY
EXERCISE	PAGE NO.	REPS	SETS	REST
MODIFIED COMPOUND SUPERSET # 1				
Biceps: Preacher Curl (alternate: Concentration Curl)	108 or 104	8–10	3	0 seconds
Triceps: Triceps Dip (alternate: Lying Triceps Extension)	118 or 120	8–10	3	60 seconds
Biceps: Hammer Curl with Rotation (alternate: Reverse E-Z Curl)	96 or 106	8–10	3	0 seconds
Triceps: Triceps Pushdown (rope) (alternate: Triceps Pushdown (bar)	114	8–10	3	60 seconds
MODIFIED COMPOUND SUPERSET # 2				
Biceps: High Cable Curl (alternate: Reverse E-Z Curl)	100 or 106	8–10	3	0 seconds
Triceps: Close Grip Bench Press (alternate: Overhead Dumbbell Triceps Extension)	116 or 110	8–10	3	60 seconds
Biceps: Dumbbell Curl (alternate: High Cable Curl)	94 or 100	8–10	3	0 seconds
Triceps: Lying E-Z Triceps Extension (alternate: Triceps Dip)	122 or 118	8–10	3	60 seconds
MODIFIED COMPOUND SUPERSET # 3				
Shoulders: Bent-Over Lateral Raise (alternate: Rear Delt on Machine)	88 or 78	8–10	3	0 seconds
Shoulders: Rotator Cuff	90	8–10	3	60 seconds
Shoulders: Cable Lateral (alternate: Dumbbell Side Lateral)	82 or 84	8–10	3	0 seconds
Shoulders: Upright Row (alternate: Military Press)	80 or 86	8–10	3	60 seconds

DAY 3 AND 6	WEDNESDAY AND SATURDAY

On Wednesdays and Saturdays you can perform the leg workout portion from the Advanced 14–Day Body Sculpting Program presented in *The Body Sculpting Bible for Men* followed by 30 minutes of cardiovascular exercise such as elliptical training, biking,running or jogging on a treadmill, or performing any other activity that will raise your heart rate to at least 220–(Your Age) x 0.75 +/– 10 beats.

WEEKS 5 & 6

SPECIAL INSTRUCTIONS:

- Perform 6–8 repetitions of each exercise for two, three or four sets as noted below.
- Perform the exercises as giant sets as prescribed below.
- Each exercise includes an alternate choice. The alternate is to be performed the second time that you hit the same muscle group on a given week. This is crucial in order to keep your body surprised and challenged and to continue to trigger muscle mass gains

DAY 1 AND 4				MONDAY AND THURSDAY
EXERCISE	PAGE NO.	REPS	SETS	REST
GIANT SET # 1				
Back: Pull–Up (Wide Grip) (alternate: Pull–Up (Close Grip)	72	6–8	4	0 seconds
Chest: Incline Dumbbell Bench Press (alternate: Incline Barbell Bench Press)	46	6–8	4	0 seconds
Back: Pull–Up (Reverse Grip) (alternate: Pull–Up (Medium Grip))	74 or 72	6–8	3	0 seconds
Chest: Chest Dip (alternate: Incline Dumbbell Bench Press)	58 or 46	6–8	3	60 seconds
GIANT SET # 2				
Chest: Barbell Bench Press (alternate: Dumbbell Bench Press)	48	6–8	4	0 seconds
Back: Row Machine (alternate: One-Arm Row)	64 or 70	6–8	4	0 seconds
Chest: Incline Cable Fly (alternate: Pullover)	52 or 66	6–8	3	0 seconds
Back: Stiff Arm Pulldown (bar) (alternate: Stiff Arm Pulldown (rope)	76	6–8	3	60 seconds
ABS WORKOUT				
Crunch on the Ball	126	20	3	15 seconds
Reverse Crunch with Legs Extended	128	20	3	15 seconds
Twist on the Ball	130	20	3	15 seconds
Crunch/Pelvic Lift Combination	138	20	3	15 seconds
Reverse Crunch	136	20	3	15 seconds
Plank with Rotation	134	20	3	15 seconds
Lower Back Extension	140	20	3	15 seconds

DAY 2 AND 5				TUESDAY AND FRIDAY
EXERCISE	**PAGE NO.**	**REPS**	**SETS**	**REST**
GIANT SET # 1				
Biceps: Preacher Curl (alternate: Concentration Curl)	108 or 104	6–8	3	0 seconds
Triceps: Triceps Dip (alternate: Lying Triceps Extension)	118 or 120	6–8	3	0 seconds
Biceps: Hammer Curl with Rotation (alternate: Reverse E-Z Curl)	96 or 106	6–8	3	0 seconds
Triceps: Triceps Pushdown (rope) (alternate: Triceps Pushdown (bar)	114	6–8	3	60 seconds
GIANT SET # 2				
Biceps: High Cable Curl (alternate: Reverse E-Z Curl)	100 or 106	6–8	3	0 seconds
Triceps: Close Grip Bench Press (alternate: Overhead Dumbbell Triceps Extension)	116 or 110	6–8	3	0 seconds
Biceps: Dumbbell Curl (alternate: High Cable Curl)	94 or 100	6–8	3	0 seconds
Triceps: Lying E-Z Triceps Extension (alternate: Triceps Dip)	122 or 118	6–8	3	60 seconds
GIANT SET # 3				
Shoulders: Bent-Over Lateral Raise (alternate: Rear Delt on Machine)	88 or 78	6–8	3	0 seconds
Shoulders: Rotator Cuff	90	6–8	3	0 seconds
Shoulders: Cable Lateral (alternate: Dumbbell Side Lateral)	82 or 84	6–8	3	0 seconds
Shoulders: Upright Row (alternate: Military Press)	80 or 86	6–8	3	60 seconds

DAY 3 AND 6	WEDNESDAY AND SATURDAY

On Wednesdays and Saturdays you can perform the leg workout portion from the Advanced 14–Day Body Sculpting Program presented in *The Body Sculpting Bible for Men* followed by 40 minutes of cardiovascular exercise such as elliptical training, biking, running or jogging on a treadmill, or performing any other activity that will raise your heart rate to at least 220–(Your Age) x 0.75 +/– 10 beats.

Daily Workout Journal

Use the log on the following page to keep track of your progress in your workouts.

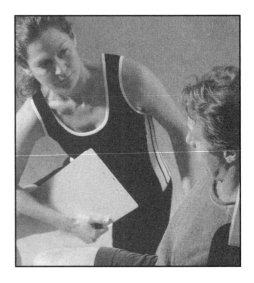

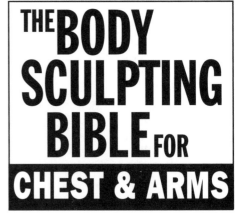

Daily Workout Journal

Week ◯ **Day** ◯

Exercise Main (Alternate)	Rest	Set 1		Set 2		Set 3		Set 4	
		Reps	Weight	Reps	Weight	Reps	Weight	Reps	Weight
Superset or Giant Set 1									
Superset or Giant Set 2									
Superset or Giant Set 3									
Superset or Giant Set 4									
Superset or Giant Set 5									
Abs									

Cardio

Cardio Activity: Notes:

Average Heart Rate:

Duration:

Use the Daily Workout Journal to keep track of your workout. Photocopy this page as many times as you need.

Appendix B

Food Charts and Nutrition

Good nutrition boils down to some simple basics:

Always try to use natural foods. Avoid using canned or prepared foods as they usually contain too much fat, sodium, and carbs.

Stay within plus or minus 10 grams of the recommended amount of carbs and proteins, plus or minus 5 grams for fats.

Always choose low–fat protein sources. Don't worry about incurring a fat deficiency since the supplements program takes care of the need for essential fatty acids. Besides, there are trace amounts of fats even in low–fat protein sources.

If you choose to include skim milk in your diet, remember that it not only has protein but also simple carbs. Therefore, count milk as both. Since the carbs in milk are simple carbs, this should only be used in the post-workout meal. However, if your schedule requires you to include more protein shakes throughout the day, and you will rely on the carbs in skim milk, add a teaspoon of flaxseed oil to the milk to slow down the release of simple carbs into the bloodstream.

Try to include fibrous carbs in at least two meals.

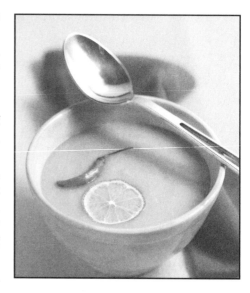

THE BODY SCULPTING BIBLE FOR CHEST & ARMS

Daily Nutrition Journal

Week ⚪ Day ⚪

	Food	Serving Size	Calories	Carbs (grams)	Protein (grams)	Fat (grams)
Meal 1						
Meal 2						
Meal 3						
Meal 4						
Meal 5						
Meal 6						
TOTAL						

Use the Daily Nutrition Journal to keep track of your diet. Photocopy the page as many times as you need.

Appendix C
Useful Resources

www.BodySculptingBible.com

A powerful resource for anyone seeking advice, knowledge, and more. Loaded with news, fitness tips, and discussion forums, this is a must-see.

www.HRFit.net

A visit here will reward you with a well-rounded bushel of information written by Hugo Rivera, ranging from how to design a workout routine to how to select or reject a food supplement.

www.JVFitness.com

This site is owned by James Villepigue, featured Fitness Trainer of *Live with Regis and Kelly*. A visit to this site will provide you with information on weight training, nutrition, supplementation, and kid/teenage training.

www.LoseFatandGainMuscle.com

For information on bodybuilding training, mass building tactics, and nutrition, this renowned site offers no-holds barred information, and brings you into the trenches of the real-deal bodybuilding lifestyle.

www.BodyTechOnline.com

The home of bodybuilding coach and fitness guru Tim Gardner who owns Body* Tech Fitness Emporium, a fine 12,000 sq. ft health and fitness club in the Florida Tampa Bay area.

www.Bodybuilding.com

Tons of free information on anything you need to know about bodybuilding and fitness, written by several experts in the industry. They also carry most supplement brands in the market selling them at a huge discount.

www.Bodybuilding.About.com

Free articles on training, nutrition, supplementation and recuperation written by Hugo Rivera, James Villepigue, and other top industry experts.

www.IronMaster.com

Home of the Quick-Lock Dumbbells, where you will find very economical, sturdy, and safe pieces of fitness equipment.

www.Powerblocks.com

A good resource for home fitness equipment.

www.FitnessFactory.com

Great place to fulfill your home gym equipment needs.

www.Prolab.com

Prolab is one of the top notch companies in the industry that carries all of the basic supplements that bodybuilders need at very affordable prices.

www.DaveDraper.com

Dave is a bodybuilding legend, winner of the Mr. America, Mr. World, and Mr. Universe titles. In his site, Dave shares his extensive knowledge in a very straight-forward, simple, and almost poetic manner.

www.MuscleBuildingDiet.com

Owned by Todd Mendelsohn, a former Mr. Central Florida who works as a nutrition/training consultant. If you want more advanced tailor made programs for bulking up then this is the place to go.